SELF-ASSESSMENT PICTURE TESTS IN VETERINARY MEDICINE

EQUINE PRACTICE

Edited by
Sue J. Dyson, MA, VetMB, DEO, FRCVS
*Equine Clinical Section, Department of
Clinical Studies, The Animal Health Trust,
Newmarket, Suffolk, England*

WOLFE PUBLISHING LTD

Copyright © Wolfe Publishing Ltd.
Published by Wolfe Publishing Ltd, 1992.
Printed by BPC Hazell, Aylesbury, England
ISBN 0 7234 1744 X

A CIP catalogue record for this book is available from the
British Library.

For full details of all Wolfe titles please write to
Wolfe Publishing Ltd, Brook House, 2–16 Torrington Place,
London WC1E 7LT, England.

PREFACE

This book is unique in its format, providing both a method of self-assessment and up-to-date information in all areas of equine medicine and surgery. Questions and answers, many of which are superbly illustrated, have been provided by leading experts in equine veterinary medicine. The questions are presented anonymously and have been mixed in order to prevent the reader making assumptions about the subject matter. They should provide a challenge to any equine practitioner and also be a stimulating method of further education: many of the answers provide information additional to that demanded in the question. Most of the questions are subdivided into sections: if problems are encountered, the reader is advised to complete each section separately; information gained from the answer to the first part of the question may help the reader to answer the remainder of the question.

I would like to thank the contributors for their tremendous efforts: without exception the task proved much more time consuming than any of us had anticipated.

ACKNOWLEDGEMENTS

Dr Long acknowledges, with gratitude, Dr J.D. Bonagura, Dr J.R. Holmes, and Mr J.A. Fraser for advice, Dr R.N. Else for performing all the post-mortem examinations, and Home of Rest for Horses, Horserace Betting Levy Board, Royal College of Veterinary Surgeons, Spencer Hill Charitable Trust, University of Edinburgh, and Diasonics Sonotron, BMS (Scotland) Ltd, for financial assistance.

LIST OF CONTRIBUTORS

W.E. Allen, MVB, PhD, Department of Veterinary Surgery and Obstetrics, Royal Veterinary College, Hatfield, Hertfordshire, England

K.C. Barnett, MA, PhD, BSc, DVOphthal, Comparative Ophthalmology Unit, Animal Health Trust, Newmarket, Suffolk, England

J.C. Brearley, MA, VetMB, DVA, Animal Health Trust, Newmarket, Suffolk, England

S.J. Dyson, MA, VetMB, DEO, Animal Health Trust, Newmarket, Suffolk, England

P.A. Harris, MA, VetMB, PhD, Animal Health Trust, Newmarket, Suffolk, England

S. Howarth, BVMS, CertVR, University of Cambridge Veterinary School, Cambridge, England

D.C. Knottenbelt, BVM & S, Division of Equine Studies, Department of Veterinary Clinical Science, University of Liverpool, Merseyside, England

A. Koterba, DVM, PhD, College of Veterinary Medicine, University of Florida, Gainesville, Florida, USA

G. Lane, BVetMed, Department of Veterinary Surgery, University of Bristol School of Veterinary Science, Bristol, England

D.P. Leadon, MA, MVB, MSc, Irish Equine Centre, Johnstown, County Kildare, Eire

K. Long, BVSc, CertVA, Veterinary Field Station, Royal (Dick) School of Veterinary Science, University of Edinburgh, Midlothian, Scotland

S. Love, BVMS, PhD, Department of Veterinary Medicine, University of Glasgow Veterinary School, Glasgow, Scotland

T.S. Mair, BVSc, PhD, DipACVIM, Department of Veterinary Medicine, University of Bristol School of Veterinary Science, Bristol, England

S.A. May, MA, VetMB, PhD, DVR, CertEO, Department of Veterinary Clinical Science, University of Liverpool, Merseyside, England

I.G. Mayhew, BVSc(Massey), Animal Health Trust, Newmarket, Suffolk, England

E.M. Milne, BVMS, PhD, MRCVS, Veterinary Field Station, Royal (Dick) School of Veterinary Medicine, University of Edinburgh, Midlothian, Scotland

R.R. Pascoe, AM, DVSc, FRCVS, FACVSc, Oakey Veterinary Hospital Pty Ltd, Oakey, Queensland, Australia

M. Schramme, B(Ghent), Department of Veterinary Surgery and Obstetrics, Royal Veterinary College, Hatfield, Hertfordshire, England

J.P. Walmesley, MA, VetMB, CertEO, Equine Veterinary Hospital, Liphook, Hampshire, England

I.M. Wright, MA, VetMB, CertEO, Animal Health Trust, Newmarket, Suffolk, England

1 A 3-year-old Thoroughbred had intermittent forelimb lameness, which was localised to the metacarpophalangeal joint; the pathology illustrated (*Figure 1*) was discovered on arthroscopic examination.
(a) What can you identify?
(b) What are the differential diagnoses?
(c) Which aspect of the joint is most commonly affected?
(d) What other diagnostic steps are important in case assessment?

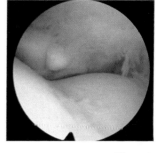

Figure 1

2 A 6-year-old event horse presented with moderate left hindlimb lameness of several weeks' duration. Lameness was accentuated by hock flexion, and not improved by subtarsal analgesia. However, perineural analgesia of the tibial and fibular (peroneal) nerves improved the lameness. Radiographs of the hock were obtained.
(a) What radiographic view is shown in *Figure 2*, and what other views would you obtain?
(b) Describe the radiographic findings.
(c) What is the likely aetiology and source of the osseous body?
(d) How would you determine its (their) significance?
(e) How can you differentiate between the lateral and medial trochlear ridges of the talus?

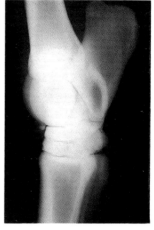

Figure 2

3 A 4-year-old child's riding pony mare developed a severe, paroxysmal cough and malodorous breath during the summer. The mare had been kept permanently at grass with one other pony for 3 months prior to the onset of coughing, and had been rested completely during this period. She had no access to hay or straw. The pony remained bright with a normal appetite, and was not dyspnoeic. There was a very slight bilateral, purulent and malodorous nasal discharge. The rectal temperature was normal, and auscultation of the chest revealed no obvious abnormalities. Submandibular lymph nodes were not enlarged.
(a) What is the most likely diagnosis, and how would you confirm it?
(b) How would you treat this condition?

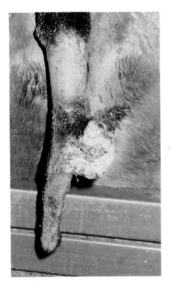

4 An 11-year-old bay gelding was found to have a tumour on the distal third of the tail (*Figure 3*). You are requested to give an opinion on treatment.
(a) What is the differential diagnosis and how would you confirm the diagnosis?
(b) What is the prognosis following surgical removal of the mass?

Figure 3

5 A 5-year-old Thoroughbred-cross gelding was found to be severely depressed 8 h after a long (7 h) road journey to an event. The mucous membranes were congested and the horse was febrile (rectal temperature 38.8°C). Shortly afterwards he showed signs of colic, which required treatment with analgesics. Three hours later he developed severe, projectile, foul-smelling diarrhoea.
(a) What disease do you suspect?
(b) What diagnostic tests would you perform?
(c) How would you treat this horse?

6 A hunter was presented for laryngeal ventriculectomy. On pre-anaesthetic examination an irregularity was noted in the pulse rate. Cardiac auscultation revealed the same abnormality in the heart rate. The ECG tracing shown in *Figure 4* was obtained.
(a) What abnormality is present?
(b) How would you determine its clinical significance?

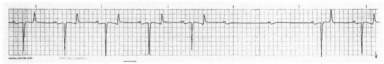

Figure 4

7 An 8-year-old show jumper gelding developed moderately severe colic signs with sudden onset. When examined 2 h after onset, pulse was 60/min, temperature 39.5°C and 5 l of fluid were refluxed from the stomach (*Figure 5*). Bowel sounds were quiet and per rectum slightly distended small intestine could be palpated. Mucous membranes were injected. Two hours later, temperature, pulse, bowel sounds and rectal findings were unchanged. A further 3 l of gastric reflux were obtained and mucous membranes were further injected with a capillary refill time of 3 s. The horse was now quiet and depressed. PCV was 46 l/l and white blood cell (WBC) count was 15×10^9/l. Peritoneal fluid was light orange coloured, total protein concentration was 35 g/l and WBC count was 1×10^9/l.

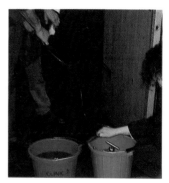

Figure 5

(a) What is your diagnosis?
(b) What action would you take?

8 A 9-year-old part-bred mare, with severe lameness of sudden onset, was referred for further investigation of a possible fracture in the hock (*Figure 6*).
(a) What is the diagnosis?
(b) What are the causes of this condition?
(c) What would be seen on hock radiographs?
(d) What might be seen on stifle radiographs?

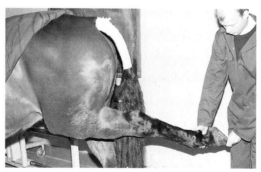

Figure 6

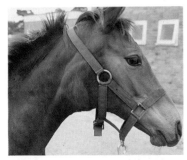

Figure 7

9 A 3-month-old Thoroughbred colt foal was not considered to be growing well. Vital signs were normal.

(a) Is the condition illustrated in *Figure 7* responsible for the failure to thrive?

(b) What is the likely aetiopathogenesis of the condition shown?

(c) What other clinical signs may be present?

10 What are the palpable features (per rectum) of a mare's reproductive tract (ovaries, uterus, cervix) in:

(a) oestrus (when does ovulation occur usually)?

(b) dioestrus?

(c) anoestrus?

(d) prolonged dioestrus?

Explain why each structure feels as it does.

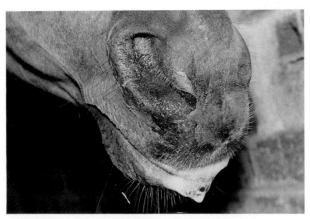

Figure 8

11 A 3-year-old pony is presented with a history of continuous colic and dysphagia of 12 h duration.

(a) Describe the signs this animal shows in *Figure 8*.

(b) What is your differential diagnosis and which condition is most likely to be present?

(c) Describe any additional clinical signs you might expect to see and the likely findings on rectal examination.

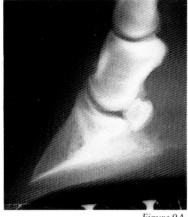

Figure 9A

Figure 9B

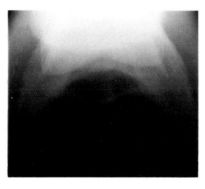

Figure 9C

12 An 8-year-old pleasure riding horse presented with mild right forelimb lameness. Lameness was accentuated on hard ground, especially when turning. Right forelimb lameness was alleviated by palmar digital nerve blocks with development of subtle left forelimb lameness. Following perineural analgesia of the palmar digital nerves of the left forelimb the horse appeared sound.

(a) What radiographic views would you obtain?
(b) Describe the radiographic features in the views shown in *Figures* 9A and B. Do you have a diagnosis?
(c) What additional information is available from *Figure 9C*?
(d) How is the view shown in *Figure 9C* obtained?
(e) What is your diagnosis and prognosis?

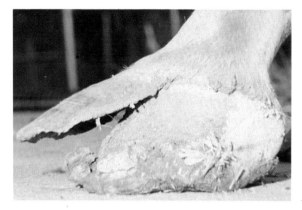

Figure 10

13 A non-pregnant mare resting in a paddock is found with a severe hoof wall separation (*Figure 10*). She is extremely lame.
(a) What are your recommendations for treatment?
(b) Will the mare be permanently lame?
(c) Would you expect that the mare will have to be always shod?

14 Do you consider that 'cystic ovaries' occur in the mare?
If the answer is yes, what are the aetiology and characteristics of the condition?
If the answer is no, what conditions of mares' ovaries suggest that they are cystic?

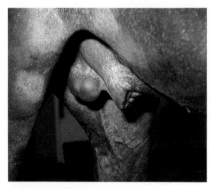

Figure 11 (courtesy of Dr P.E. Holt, University of Bristol)

15 A 3-year-old gelding is presented 8 months following castration, for the investigation of a suspected inguinal hernia (*Figure 11*).
(a) What is your differential diagnosis?
(b) What is the most likely aetiology?
(c) What other clinical findings may be present?
(d) How would you manage this case?
(e) What is the prognosis?

16 The unilateral clinical sign shown in *Figure 12* had persisted for several months with little change. The animal had been under treatment for navicular disease.

(a) List the most likely conditions which present with this sign.

(b) What further diagnostic measures should be employed and how might the various conditions be identified from these?

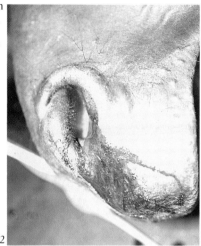

Figure 12

17 A 2-year-old pony mare developed sudden-onset, severe watery diarrhoea in early January (*Figure 13*). The pony had been kept permanently at pasture with a group of other horses since birth. She was given supplementary feeding during the winter, and was wormed regularly at 8-week intervals (last wormed 5 days prior to the onset of illness). Since the onset of diarrhoea 3 days previously, she had lost a considerable amount of weight, and had developed ventral oedema. On clinical examination the pony was found to be depressed and slightly dehydrated; her rectal temperature was 37.7°C. A faeces sample yielded a profuse growth of *Salmonella typhimurium* and no worm eggs. Haematological examination revealed a PCV of 50 l/l and a mild leucocytosis (WBC 14.3×10^9/l) with neutrophilia (PMN 9.8×10^9/l). Serum biochemistry revealed hypoalbuminaemia (albumin 2.1 g/dl).

(a) What condition do you suspect, and how would you confirm your diagnosis?

(b) What treatment would you advise?

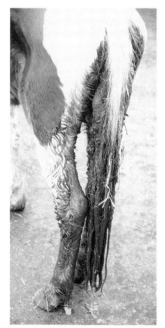

Figure 13

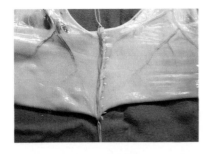

Figure 14A. Everting mattress suture.

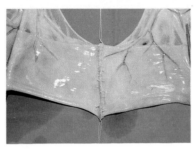

Figure 14B. Opposing simple interrupted suture.

18 Exploratory laparotomy reveals a strangulation of 1.5 m (5 feet) of jejunum by a pedunculated lipoma in a horse. After reduction you need to decide whether the strangulated bowel segment requires resection and anastomosis.

(a) Which factors will help you assess the viability of the segment, and therefore the necessity for resection?

(b) 2.15 m (7 feet) of jejunum need resecting. Would you elect to create an end-to-end anastomosis or side-to-side anastomosis between the transected ends of jejunum? Explain why.

(c) The success of the intestinal anastomosis depends greatly on the use of an appropriate suture pattern that minimises the incidence of adhesions, stenosis and leakage. Make and explain your choice from the list below:

- Single-layer everting suture (e.g. vertical mattress) (*Figure 14A*).
- Single-layer opposing suture (e.g. simple interrupted) (*Figure 14B*).
- Single-layer inverting suture (e.g. interrupted Lembert) (*Figure 14C*).
- Double-layer inverting closure (opposing layer plus inverting layer) (*Figure 14D*).

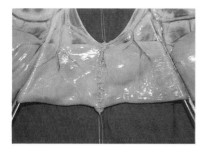 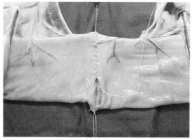

Figure 14C. Inverted interrupted Lembert suture.

Figure 14D. Double-layer inverting closure (simple interrupted plus continuous Lembert).

(d) What suture material would you use for intestinal anastomosis? Why?
- Chromic catgut.
- Catgut.
- Polyglycolic acid.
- Polyglactin 910.
- PDS suture.
- Braided polyester.
- Monofilament nylon.

(e) Why are stapling devices considered inappropriate for small intestinal end-to-end anastomosis?

19 The Doppler study in *Figure 15* was obtained from a 7-year-old dressage horse with a grade 3/6 systolic murmur over the right hemithorax. The murmur was localised at the fourth intercostal space just below the heart base. The murmur was auscultated during a routine examination prior to vaccination.

(a) What is your diagnosis?
(b) How would you assess its severity?
(c) Is this condition likely to affect the animal's performance?

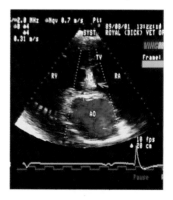

Figure 15. Right ventricle (RV); tricuspid valve (TV); aortic valve (AO); right atrium (RA).

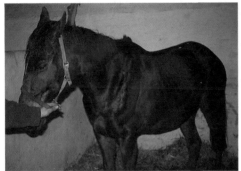

Figure 16A   Figure 16B

20 An 11-year-old eventer gelding (*Figure 16A*) had had recurrent bouts of mild colic for 1 week. Its abdomen was mildly distended and guarded when palpated. Its temperature was 39°C, pulse 45/min, borborygmus was depressed; mucous membranes were injected. Faeces were dry and scanty and per rectum no abnormalities were detected although manipulation of the rectum felt restricted. No gastric reflux was obtained. Haematological parameters were as follows: PCV 42 l/l; TP 75 g/l; albumin 21 g/l; globulin 54 g/l; fibrinogen 5.0 g/l; WBC 10×10^9/l; PMN 6.3×10^9/l with a left shift. Peritoneal fluid (*Figure 16B*); nucleated cell count 14×10^9/l with large numbers of macrophages and polymorphonuclear leucocytes; total protein 40 g/l.
(a) What is your diagnosis?
(b) Which of the above parameters are the most reliable for diagnosing this case?
(c) How would you treat this gelding?

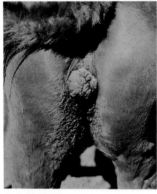

Figure 17

21 A 17-year-old mare is presented with a variety of lesions around the tail hair, anus and vulva (*Figure 17*).
(a) What could be causing the tail problem?
(b) What is the most likely condition on the lower vulvar commissure?
(c) Can surgery correct the second condition?

14

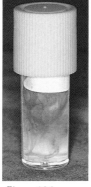

Figure 18A

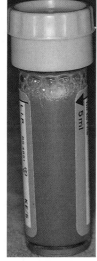

Figure 18B

22 What is the interpretation of the gross appearance of synovial fluid samples A (*Figure 18A*) and B (*Figure 18B*)? What further measures would you take with these cases?

23 A 5-year-old Dutch Warmblood gelding presented with left hindlimb lameness of several weeks' duration. Lameness was markedly accentuated by hock flexion.
(a) What radiographic views would you obtain?
(b) What views are seen in *Figure 19A* and *B*? Describe the radiographic features in both views.
(c) What additional views might you obtain?
(d) How would you determine the significance of the radiographic abnormalities?
(e) What is the likely aetiology?

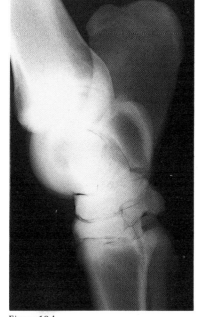

Figure 19A

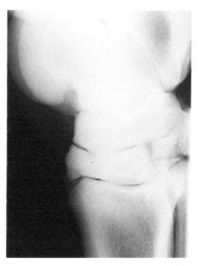

Figure 19B

24 How might endometritis, caused by opportunistic pathogens, be:
(a) Suspected?
(b) Diagnosed?
(c) Prevented?
(d) Treated.

25 A 12-hour-old term Thoroughbred filly is found down in the stall, thrashing and seizuring. The birth process was observed to be normal, and the foal had stood and nursed within 2 h of birth. The body temperature is now 40.5°C, the heart rate 160 beats/min, the respiratory rate 80 breaths/min and shallow, and mucous membranes are a muddy blue colour.
(a) What is your immediate therapy?
(b) What diagnostic tests are indicated?
(c) What are the most likely differential diagnoses?
(d) What is your prognosis for the recovery of this foal, based on the most likely differential diagnosis?

26 (a) Is the retina shown in *Figure 20* (from an 8-year-old Thoroughbred) normal?
(b) What are the distinguishing ophthalmoscopic features in *Figure 20*?

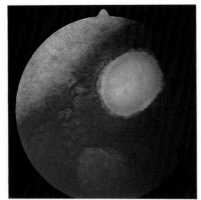

Figure 20

27 A 10-year-old three-day event gelding presented with an intermittent right forelimb lameness of 3 years' duration. Lameness had tended to be barely detectable to slight with normal work, including one-day events, but after each three-day event deteriorated. It had previously resolved with rest but following the last three-day event had persisted. The horse tended to point the right forelimb at rest. There was slight enlargement on the palmar aspect of the pastern. Lameness was improved but not alleviated by perineural analgesia of the palmar digital

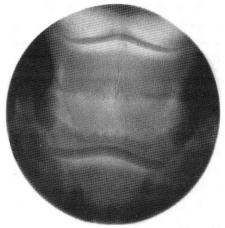

Figure 21

nerves. A radiograph of the right front foot was obtained (*Figure 21*).
(a) What radiographic views would you obtain?
(b) Describe the radiographic findings in *Figure 21*.
(c) How would you interpret these?
(d) What additional diagnostic tests would you perform?

28 The procedure shown in *Figure 22* followed palmar digital nerve blocks.
(a) What causes of lameness is this animal unlikely to be suffering from?
(b) What procedure is being undertaken?
(c) If this has no effect on the problem, what is the clinician likely to do next?

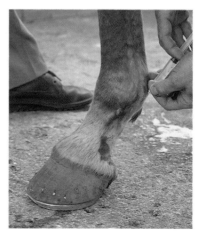

Figure 22

29 (a) What clinical signs can you identify in *Figure 23*?
(b) What is the diagnosis?
(c) What factors may affect the prognosis?

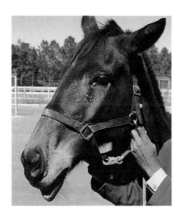

Figure 23

30 An 11-year-old mare has had a 9-week history of weight loss and lethargy. The submandibular lymph nodes and parotid glands had become grossly enlarged (*Figure 24*). There was an early period of pyrexia (rectal temperature 39.9°C), which led to an initial diagnosis of respiratory infection due to *Streptococcus equi* (strangles). In the last few weeks she has developed a stridulous respiratory noise, and has become mildly dysphagic. Endoscopic examination of the upper airways has shown multiple nodular swellings of the nasopharyngeal and laryngeal mucosa.
(a) What is the differential diagnosis?
(b) What further diagnostic procedures would you perform?

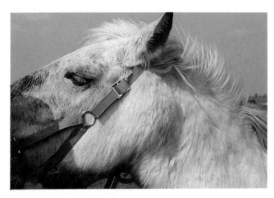

Figure 24

31 A severe ringbark lesion of the proximal metatarsus has removed a large area of skin (*Figure 25*). Assuming that the blood supply to the distal limb is intact, and that no joint, tendon or ligament is involved:
(a) What treatment should be given?
(b) In a show horse, from where would you obtain a donor graft and why?

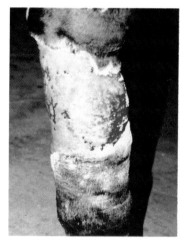

Figure 25

32 An 11-year-old hunter gelding had spasms of colic all day and passed only small amounts of faeces. Hyoscine-N-butylbromide and dipyrone (Buscopan compositum) relieved the pain but colic started again as the drugs wore off. The heart rate was 44 beats/min, PCV 45%, mucous membranes of normal appearance and gut sounds reduced. Paracentesis produced frank blood. On rectal examination (*Figure 26*) the spleen was displaced ventrally and caudally. A succession of tight bands was felt to extend transversely through the abdominal cavity, converging upward, forward and to the left. They seemed abnormally anchored at the level of the left kidney. The tightly stretched nephrosplenic ligament could not be reached from the dorsal edge of the spleen, but was felt to extend vertically downward from the caudal edge of the left kidney. The large colon was distended with gas and impacted.

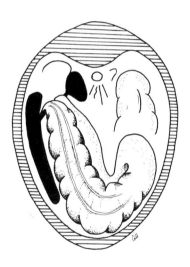

Figure 26. Rectal findings.

(a) What is your diagnosis?
(b) What treatment would you advise?
(c) Is there another option? Describe the different steps of this conservative approach.
(d) What is your prognosis?
(e) Why did paracentesis yield frank blood?

33 An owner requests information on protein requirements for growth and exercise.
(a) How much protein should you advise to be fed?
(b) Would feeding excess be harmful?
(c) Does it matter what the source of the protein is?
(d) Can the horse utilise non-protein nitrogen?

34 A 3-year-old Thoroughbred gelding has developed a cough and bilateral, malodorous nasal discharge, which is intermittently blood tinged. The horse is pyrexic (rectal temperature 39.4°C) and has moderate inspiratory and expiratory dyspnoea. Endoscopic examination showed a purulent discharge draining from the right bronchial tree. Thoracic radiographs revealed a lesion in the dorsocaudal lung field (*Figure 27*).
(a) What is the likely diagnosis?
(b) How would you investigate the case further?

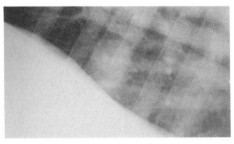

Figure 27

35 A gelding is presented with colic and scrotal swelling 6 h after a standing open castration (*Figure 28*).
(a) What is your diagnosis?
(b) What immediate surgical considerations must be addressed?
(c) How may this condition have been prevented?

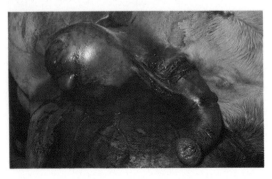

Figure 28 (courtesy of Dr P.E. Holt, University of Bristol)

Figure 29

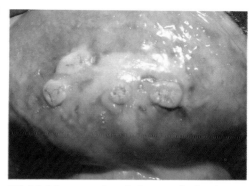

36 (a) How may these lesions on the lip shown in *Figure 29* be explained?
(b) Are they associated with any significant pathological condition?

37 A 2-year-old Thoroughbred colt developed dyspnoea, a harsh inspiratory noise and a sporadic cough soon after he was brought into work. You examined the horse 6 months after the onset of clinical signs, when a pronounced, harsh 'roaring' inspiratory noise was present at rest, and vibrations were palpable over the entire cervical trachea. Endoscopy revealed an excess of mucus in the upper trachea, and an irregular dorsoventral constriction, which extended for a distance of 15 cm, at the level of the thoracic inlet (*Figure 30*). The trachea and major bronchi distal to this area appeared normal.
(a) What is the likely nature of this lesion?
(b) Is any treatment possible?

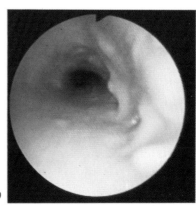

Figure 30

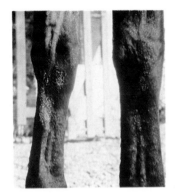

38 (a) What are the yellow structures present on the skin of the forelimb of the horse shown in *Figure 31*?
(b) What is their pathogenic significance?
(c) How would you manage this condition?

Figure 31

39 A 5-year-old Clydesdale gelding is presented with a papillomatous area with a small granulating non-healing sore on the non-pigmented skin of the upper lip (*Figure 32*).
(a) What is the differential diagnosis?
(b) How would you confirm your diagnosis?

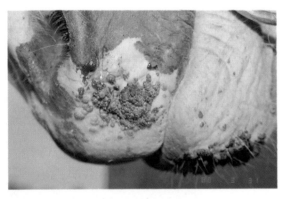

Figure 32

40 During palpation per rectum of an ovary, the mare tenses the muscles of her flank and slowly lifts the hind leg on the side of the ovary being examined. What is the likely cause of this behaviour?

Figure 33

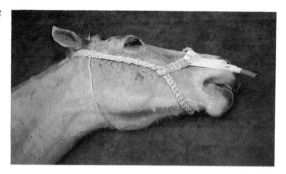

41 The horse shown in *Figure 33* has just been placed in recovery after a 60-min duration anaesthetic in dorsal recumbency.
(a) What is illustrated here?
(b) Give two causes of the possible condition that is being treated.

42 A yearling colt presented with a stiff hindlimb gait and bilateral distension of the femoropatellar joints. Radiographic examination revealed an irregularly flattened contour to the lateral trochlear ridge of the femur with overlying islands of mineralised tissue. *Figure 34* shows the arthroscopic appearance of the lateral trochlear ridge.
(a) What is your diagnosis?
(b) What is the current treatment of choice?
(c) What is the rationale for this treatment?

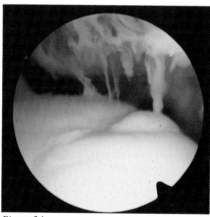

Figure 34

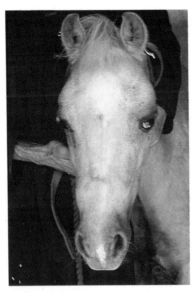

Figure 35

43 The sign illustrated in *Figure 35* developed slowly over several months.
(a) Describe the clinical features.
(b) What conditions might be responsible?
(c) What further investigations may be used to clarify the type of lesion responsible?.

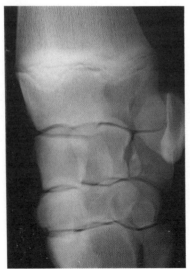

Figure 36

44 A 7-month-old Thoroughbred colt presented with left forelimb lameness of several weeks' duration. The lameness was variable in degree, both within and between exercise periods. The left front foot was narrower and more upright than the right. Subcarpal analgesia failed to improve the lameness. Radiographs of the carpus were obtained.
(a) What view is shown in *Figure 36*? What other views would you obtain?
(b) Describe the radiographic features.
(c) How would you determine their significance?

45 Clinical and laboratory findings suggest that a horse has impairment of hepatic function and that a liver biopsy is indicated.
(a) What type of biopsy needle is shown in *Figure 37*?
(b) What is (are) the site(s) for liver biopsy in equines?
(c) What important factors must be considered before carrying out the biopsy procedure?

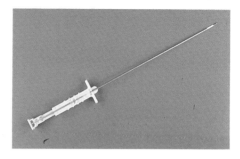

Figure 37

46 (a) Which bacteria commonly cause endometritis in mares and what factors contribute to the aetiology?
(b) Culture of a uterine swab on blood agar resulted in a pure growth of domed, non-pigmented colonies which look like staphylococci. *Figure 38A* shows the result of staining a smear of one of the colonies using Diff Quik. What is your diagnosis?
(c) Routine ultrasound examination of a hunter mare arriving at stud for covering revealed fluid in the uterus. This was aspirated and found to be mucoid in consistency. Culture on blood agar produced an extensive fluffy growth; a photomicrograph (stained with lactophenol cotton blue) is shown in *Figure 38B*.
What is your diagnosis?

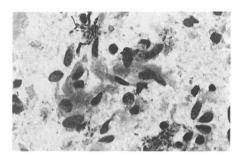

Figure 38A

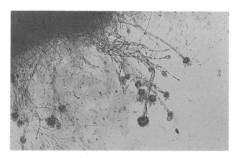

Figure 38B

Figure 39

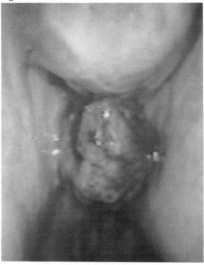

47 *Figure 39* illustrates the endoscopic view of the caudal nasal area of an aged hunter which has shown intermittent right-sided epistaxis for several months.
(a) What is the lesion?
(b) How can the lesion be treated?
(c) What is the prognosis?

48 The 11-month-old Thoroughbred colt, illustrated in *Figure 40A* and *B*, normal at birth, now has difficulty walking.
(a) How long is it likely that this animal has been affected?
(b) In which limb is the primary problem?
(c) What is the differential diagnosis for the cause of the primary problem?
(d) What is the secondary problem, and why has it developed?

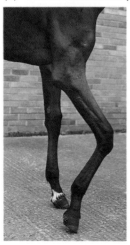

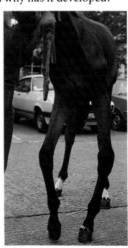

Figure 40A

Figure 40B

49 A 17-year-old cob mare had been suffering repeated bouts of colic over a 9-month period. The bouts of pain had become progressively more frequent and severe. Rectal examination during these bouts revealed moderately distended loops of small intestine, but between bouts no abnormality could be detected. An exploratory laparotomy revealed three, firm, annular thickenings of the jejunum; no other abnormalities were detected, other than a slight enlargement of many of the mesenteric lymph nodes.
(a) What is the likely nature of these lesions?
(b) What is the prognosis?

50 (a) What clinical signs are apparent in the animal shown in *Figure 41*?
(b) Several horses in the stable yard had presented with lameness and inappetence. Are the signs in this animal likely to be found in others in the yard?
(c) What additional diagnostic test(s) might you employ?

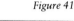

Figure 41

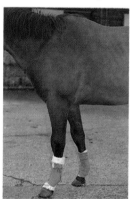

51 An infected splint bone fracture was removed surgically from a 7-year-old hunter gelding. The next day the gelding showed mild signs of abdominal discomfort. Both the animal's appetite and faecal output were reduced. The heart rate was 48 beats/min, few gut sounds were present and mucous membranes were normal.

Rectal examination revealed the presence of a large, firm but indentable mass, with a distinct band running in a dorsoventral direction forward, in the right half of the abdomen (*Figure 42*). The left side of the abdomen was empty. Discomfort was easily controlled with analgesics but returned a few hours after injection. On rectal examination the mass was now of a harder consistency.
(a) What is the likely diagnosis?
(b) What action would you advise?
(c) What are the risks of conservative management?
(d) What are the surgical alternatives?

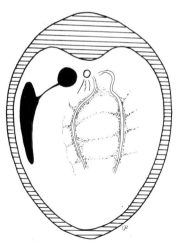

Figure 42. Rectal findings.

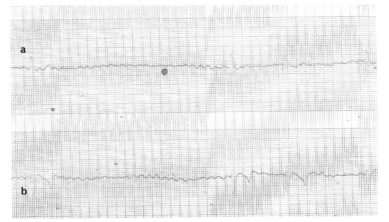

Figure 43A. (a) lead Z;
(b) lead Y; paper speed,
25 mm/sec.

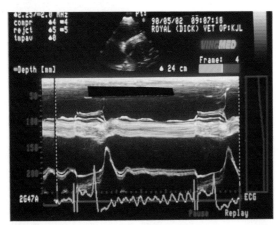

Figure 43B

52 A 9-year-old hunter was presented with a history of epistaxis and reduced performance. Endoscopy of the upper and lower respiratory tract revealed no abnormalities.

(a) What does the ECG in *Figure 43A* reveal?

(b) What does the M-mode echocardiogram of the mitral valve show (*Figure 43B*)?

(c) How might this condition be treated?

(d) What further information would you require to decide whether treatment would be advisable or successful?

53 *Figure 44* is the endoscopic view of the larynx of a 4-year-old hurdler which has developed stridulous respiratory noises at exercise during the past month having previously been normal.
(a) What is the cause of the stridor?
(b) What treatment would you advise?

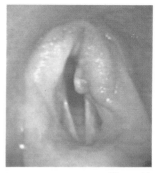

Figure 44

54 A mare is presented with ventral oedema (*Figure 45*) 3 months after a hunting accident where she became straddled over a gate.
(a) What is your diagnosis and how might you confirm it?
(b) What surgical technique would be appropriate for treatment?
(c) What materials would you use and why?

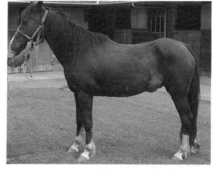

Figure 45 (courtesy of Dr P.E. Holt, University of Bristol)

Figure 46

55 Marked weight loss was the main complaint in the 7-year-old gelding shown in *Figure 46*.
(a) How can the distribution of the oedema be explained?
(b) What changes might be expected in the body temperature of this case?

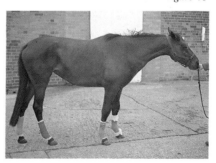

Figure 47

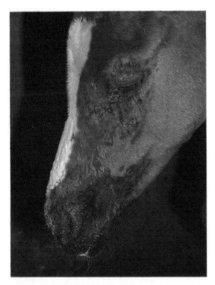

56 A 4-week-old Arabian colt foal has had an 8-day history of chronic diarrhoea, dyspnoea, bilateral purulent nasal discharge, intermittent pyrexia (rectal temperature up to 38.9°C), alopecia and crusting skin lesions, and weight loss (*Figure 47*). The foal has already been treated with a variety of antibiotics, oral fluid and electrolyte solutions, and oral kaolin/pectin mixtures. The foal was born normally at full term, and had sucked frequently within 2 h of birth. Thoracic radiographs showed mild consolidation of the ventral lung fields. Results of some of the clinicopathological tests are summarised below:

	Foal	Normal
PCV (%)	32	30–42
WBC × 10^9/l	8.8	5.9–8.7
Neutrophils × 10^9/l	7.8	1.1–7.5
Lymphocytes × 10^9/l	0.2	0.8–4.8

Faecal examination: numerous cryptosporidial oocysts
Transtracheal aspirate culture: *Streptococcus zooepidemicus*
Skin scrape examination: *Dermatophilus congolensis*

(a) What is the likely diagnosis, and how can this be confirmed?
(b) Discuss the aetiology of the various clinical features of the case?

57 What is the rationale for obtaining a plasma sample for progesterone determination in a non-pregnant mare?

58 A 12-year-old brood mare is lame. Originally, she had sustained a severe wire cut to the coronary band and bulb of the heel. This had healed and the mare was supposedly doing well when lameness reoccurred with the appearance of a granulating mass of tissue over the heel (*Figure 48*).
(a) What conditions could be present?
(b) What treatments could be used?
(c) How successful are they likely to be?

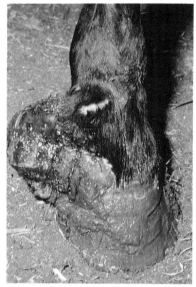

Figure 48

Figure 49

59 (a) Is the retina shown in *Figure 49* (from a 12-year-old hunter) normal?
(b) What are the distinguishing ophthalmoscopic features?

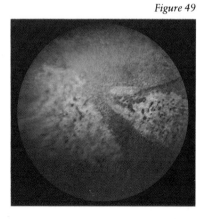

31

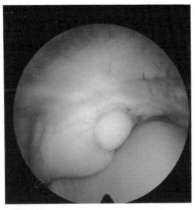

Figure 50

60 The arthroscopic appearance of osteochondritis dissecans of the medial malleolus of the tibia in a yearling is illustrated in *Figure 50*.
(a) Which radiographic projection(s) is/are likely to have predicted the presence of this lesion?
(b) List, in descending order of incidence, the sites of osteochondritis dissecans recorded in the tarsocrural joint.

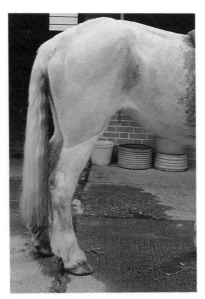

Figure 51

61 The horse illustrated in *Figure 51* had recovered well some 3 weeks previously from an upper respiratory tract infection. The tail is flaccid and urine overflow and faecal contamination have soiled the hocks and tail. The hindquarters are poorly muscled.
(a) What is your differential diagnosis?
(b) Are these clinical signs related to the previous history?
(c) What is the prognosis for this horse?

62 A 4-year-old pony mare was presented with a 5-week history of rapid weight loss, depression and ventral oedema (*Figure 52*). Her appetite was capricious, and faecal consistency normal. Clinical examination was unremarkable other than confirming poor condition and ventral oedema. Routine haematology was normal, and a serum biochemistry profile revealed hypoproteinaemia and hypoalbuminaemia (albumin 14.l g/l), and elevated alkaline phosphatase (SAP 1130 u/l); all other liver enzymes (SDH, GLDH, GGT, AST), and urea and creatinine were normal. A bromosulphthalein (BSP) clearance test was normal. Urinalysis and peritoneal fluid analysis were normal.

(a) What are your conclusions about this case?

(b) What further diagnostic tests would you perform?

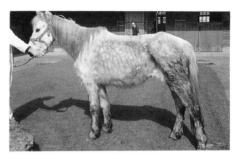

Figure 52

63 *Figure 53* shows the pattern of proteins separated by electrophoresis of a serum sample taken from a 15-year-old riding horse with a history of diarrhoea and weight loss of 2 month's duration.

(a) What are the abnormalities present on the tracing?

(b) What is the likely diagnosis?

(c) How would you confirm the diagnosis?

(d) What treatment would you recommend and what is the prognosis for this case?

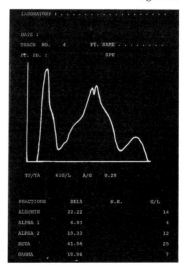

Figure 53

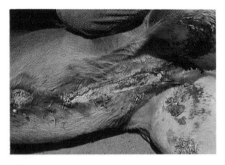

64 An abdominal wound following surgery for a ruptured urachus with urinary discharge subcutaneously has failed to heal (*Figure 54*).
(a) How would you manage this wound in a 14-day-old foal?
(b) What is the risk of eventration occurring?

Figure 54

65 A 3-year-old Irish draught stallion returned from service duties and had a sudden bout of severe colic. When examined 4 h later, the animal was in continuous pain, had a heart rate of 80 beats/min and red, injected mucous membranes. No bowel sounds could be heard on auscultation. On palpation both testicles were found to be present but they seemed to be of different sizes. Normal peritoneal fluid was retrieved on paracentesis.
(a) What might you find on rectal examination?
(b) What is your diagnosis?
(c) Why was the peritoneal fluid normal?
(d) What treatment would you advise?

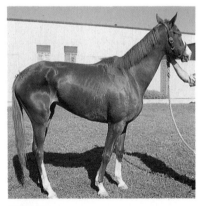

66 A 2-year-old Thoroughbred filly in training, shown in *Figure 55*, developed atrophy of the right quadriceps muscles with no detectable gait abnormality. After 1 month, atrophy of the longissimus lumborum from L2 to L6 developed and the filly became paraparetic and ataxic, showing the worst symptoms on the right side. What is:
(a) The site of the lesion?
(b) The most probable cause of this disease?
(c) The current therapy for this disease?

Figure 55

67 The pony in *Figure 56* had received an 'intramuscular' injection in the lower third of the neck.
(a) What diagnostic procedures would be indicated in the investigation of this swelling?
(b) What possible immediate consequences might occur?
(c) What possible long-term complications might arise?

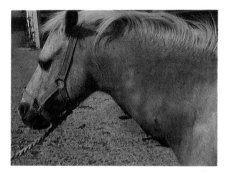

Figure 56

68 An 11-month-old colt has been growing rapidly since weaning.
(a) What clinical signs are shown in *Figure 57*?
(b) Are these problems linked?
(c) What are the most likely causes of the clinical signs?
(d) What management advice should be given to the owner?

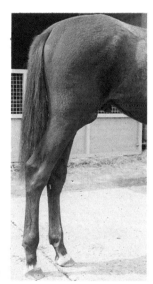

Figure 57

69 (a) What organisms are considered to cause venereal disease in horses?
(b) What are the clinical signs in stallions and mares?
(c) How can the spread of these conditions be minimised?

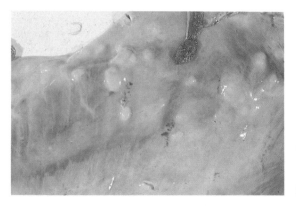

Figure 58

70 The appearance of the peritoneum of the body wall in a horse that was humanely destroyed following a 5-month illness of recurrent colic and chronic weight loss is illustrated in *Figure 58*.
(a) What are the lesions shown?
(b) Are these lesions likely to be associated with the clinical signs?

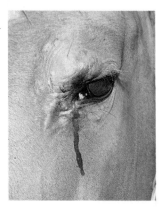

Figure 59

71 A 5-year-old brood mare is presented with epiphora and a hairless, slightly swollen upper eyelid which contains several shot-like nodules under the skin (*Figure 59*). The owner requests your advice.
(a) What is the differential diagnosis?
(b) How could you confirm your diagnosis?
(c) What are the dangers in this?
(d) How can this condition be treated?

72 Some difficulty had been experienced in placing an intravenous catheter; when attempts were discontinued the catheter was withdrawn and its appearance is shown in *Figure 60*.
(a) How was this caused?
(b) What could have been the consequence if attempts at placement had persisted?

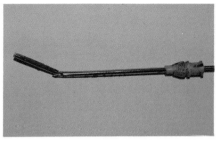

Figure 60

73 Examination of an ovary, per rectum, is proving difficult because, although the ovary has been located and touched with the fingertips, its contours cannot be palpated clearly; why?

74 The yearling colt shown in *Figure 61* has an umbilical swelling.
(a) How may such lesions be classified?
(b) What further information will influence the surgical approach to this animal?
(c) What surgical techniques may be used to treat this condition?
(d) What ethical considerations are relevant to this condition?

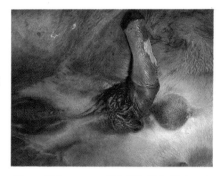

Figure 61 (courtesy of Dr P.E. Holt, University of Bristol)

75 What is the significance of measuring oestrone sulphate in the blood of pregnant mares? How is this related to the 'urine test'?

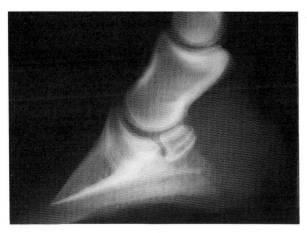

Figure 62A

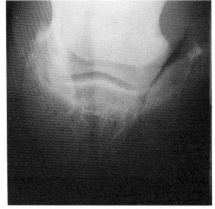

Figure 62B

76 A 9-year-old hunter gelding presented with an acute onset of severe right forelimb lameness. There was a slight increase in the amplitude of the pulses in the digital vessels. Pressure applied to the medial aspect of the midsole with hoof testers caused pain. Exploration of the foot was otherwise negative. No change developed after poulticing for 3 days. Perineural analgesia of the palmar (abaxial sesamoid) nerves improved but by no means alleviated the lameness.

Figure 62C

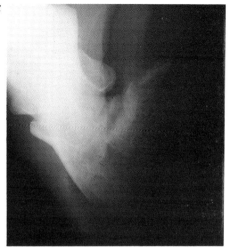

Figure 62D

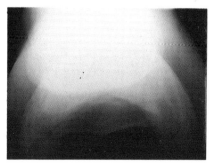

(a) What radiographic views would you obtain?
(b) Describe the radiographic features in *Figure 62 A–C*.
(c) What additional view(s) would you obtain?
(d) Describe the radiographic features in *Figure 62D*. What is your diagnosis, treatment and prognosis?

Figure 63

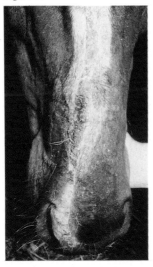

77 A 10-year-old hunter has developed a painful dermatitis, affecting the area over the nasal bones (illustrated in *Figure 63*) and the non-pigmented areas below the fetlock joints, over a period of 4 weeks. Weight loss and lethargy has been noticed for the past 3 months.
(a) What type of dermatitis is likely to be present and what are the possible causes?
(b) What is the pathogenesis of this dermatitis?

78 A 10-year-old pony gelding was presented with a 1-week history of sudden onset of dyspnoea and tachypnoea. A plaque of subcutaneous oedema had developed over the ventral sternum 2 days prior to the examination (*Figure 64*). Clinical examination revealed tachypnoea (respiratory rate 32/min) with marked inspiratory and expiratory dyspnoea. Auscultation of both sides of the thorax revealed crackling and wheezing sounds dorsally, but muffling of the lung sounds in the ventral half of the chest. Percussion of the thorax revealed significant dullness ventrally.
(a) What is the likely cause of the dyspnoea?
(b) What is the differential diagnosis and how would you investigate the case further?

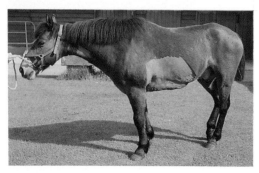

Figure 64

79 *Figure 65* shows the endoscopic finding in a 4-year-old cob which had shown a tendency to vibrant inspiratory sounds at exercise ever since it was broken in. What abnormalities can you see and what advice would you give?

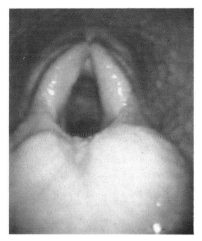

Figure 65

80 Hock wounds are difficult to treat. A child's pony is presented with a chronic wound (*Figure 66*).
(a) The owner's finances are limited. What treatment would you advise?
(b) How long might it take to heal?
(c) Will there be any after-effects?

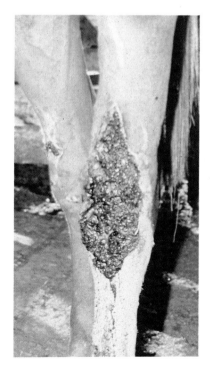

Figure 66

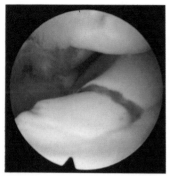

Figure 67

81 A 5-year-old hurdler finished a race acutely lame. The limb was bandaged but next day marked metacarpophalangeal joint distension was evident and fracture of the medial proximal sesamoid bone was diagnosed radiographically. The arthroscopic appearance of the fracture is shown in *Figure 67*.

(a) What is the aetiology of such fractures?

(b) What other technique(s) may be employed to obtain useful prognostic information?

(c) What are the generally quoted criteria for the removal of such fragments?

82 The post-mortem appearance of the colonic mucosa from a 3-year-old Thoroughbred filly that died 1 week after developing sudden-onset diarrhoea in March is illustrated in *Figure 68*. The animal had a poor appetite during the illness and was observed to have low grade abdominal pain on several occasions. No veterinary advice was sought but the owner requested a post-mortem examination of the animal, which was performed 24 h following its death.

(a) What is the diagnosis?

(b) What additional procedures would help to confirm this diagnosis?

(c) What are the important aspects of the pathogenesis of this condition?

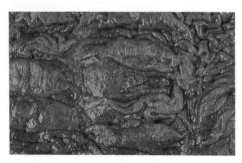

Figure 68

83 (a) You are presented with a 2-year-old Arab filly because a pink, balloon-like structure is sometimes seen protruding between the vulval lips, particularly when she lies down or is urinating. What is your diagnosis? How would you confirm this and treat the condition?
(b) You are called to see a mare which has foaled during the night unobserved. There is a longitudinal vestibulorectal tear extending about 15 cm cranially from the perineum. What has caused the lesion? What is your initial advice and treatment and how would you manage the case in the long term?

84 Venous blood sample evacuated container systems vary in the colour of the tube stopper, and in tube contents. Indicate the appropriate usage of *stopper colours* violet, blue, black, grey, red and green for the *tube contents* EDTA, sodium citrate (3.8%), sodium citrate (3.1%), sodium fluoride–potassium oxalate, plain (no anticoagulant), and lithium heparin.

85 *Figure 69* is a post post-mortem photograph of the mitral valve of a 4-year-old mare.
(a) What is the likely diagnosis?
(b) What clinical features may have been seen and how would you make this diagnosis in life?
(c) How would you treat this condition?
(d) What factors would determine the likely outcome?

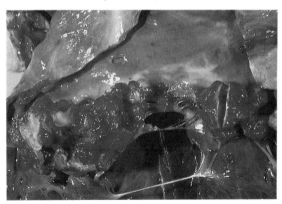

Figure 69

Figure 70

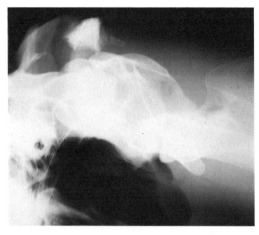

86 A horse grazing with others is found one morning unable to raise its head from the ground. It is able to walk with normal coordination and shows no obvious neurological deficiency. A plain lateral radiograph (*Figure 70*) was obtained with the horse conscious. What is your diagnosis and what measures would you take to treat the horse?

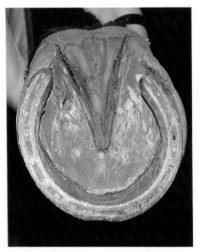

Figure 71

87 (a) Does the horse whose foot is illustrated in *Figure 71* have a problem?
(b) What advice is indicated?

Figure 72

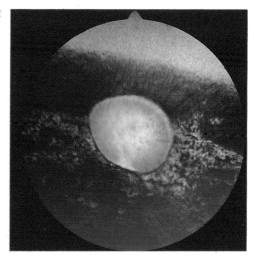

88 (a) Is the retina illustrated in *Figure 72* (from a 7-year-old hunter) normal?
(b) What are the distinguishing ophthalmoscopic features?

Figure 73

89 A 3-year-old mare was noticed to have a warty eruption with loss of hair (*Figure 73*). It has been present for over 12 months and the owner requests your advice.
(a) What is the probable cause?
(b) Is it likely to be infectious to other horses?
(c) Would you advise surgical excision?
(d) What percentage would you expect to be cured with surgery alone?

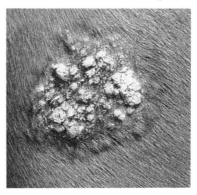

45

Figure 74

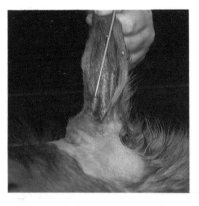

90 A yearling is presented with a discharging sinus at the rostral margin of the base of the pinna. *Figure 74* shows a metal seeker introduced into the sinus tract. What is your diagnosis and what further investigation should be performed? What treatment is indicated?

91 A 6-year-old hunter gelding with a 9-day history of dullness, lethargy, inappetence, weight loss and mild diarrhoea, was examined. The horse also showed signs of chronic, low grade abdominal pain (lying down a lot, turning to look at flanks, yawning, etc.), and had demonstrated intermittent pyrexia (rectal temperature as high as 40.0°C) since the onset of illness. Rectal examination was unremarkable. Abdominal paracentesis yielded cloudy, red-brown fluid (*Figure 75*).

Significant clinical pathological abnormalities included the following: WBC, $18.5 \times 10^9/l$; PMN, $15.0 \times 10^9/l$; bands, $1.1 \times 10^9/l$; plasma fibrinogen, 7.5 g/l; peritoneal fluid nucleated cell count, $85.4 \times 10^9/l$; PMN, $84.7 \times 10^9/l$ (toxic and pyknotic neutrophils were also identified).
(a) What is the diagnosis?
(b) What are the possible underlying causes?
(c) How would you treat this horse?

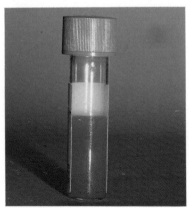

Figure 75

92 A 7-year-old Thoroughbred mare had a vague history of exercise intolerance, intermittent fever (up to 40.6°C), tachypnoea (respiratory rate up to 60/min at rest) and hindlimb oedema over a 6-week period. The mucous membranes, including the vulva, were pale with numerous petechial and ecchymotic haemorrhages (*Figure 76*). Haematological examination revealed anaemia (PCV, 16%; RBC, 3.10 × 10^{12}/l; Hb, 5.0 g/dl), neutropenia (PMN, 0.10 × 10^9/l), lymphocytosis (lymphocyte count, 9.14 × 10^9/l) and thrombocytopenia (platelet count, 35 × 10^9/l). What is the likely diagnosis, and how would you confirm it?

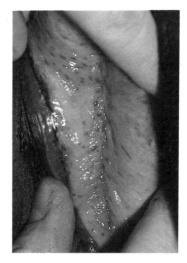

Figure 76

93 The oesophagus shown in *Figure 77* was obtained from a 5-year-old mare which had been destroyed due to chronic severe colic.
(a) What is the likely cause of the lesions illustrated?
(b) What is the most likely underlying disease to account for both colic and these lesions?
(c) What post-mortem material may enable a definitive diagnosis to be established?
(d) Has the owner any cause for concern for the other horses on the property?

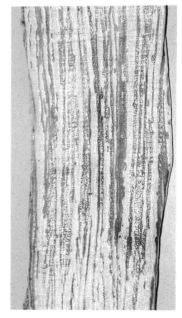

Figure 77

94 Granulosa cell tumours:
(a) Affect mares of what age range usually?
(b) Cause what clinical signs?
(c) Are diagnosed by?
(d) Are best treated by?
(e) What prognosis can be given?

95 The blood biochemical and haematological results in *Table 1* were obtained from a pregnant, 10-year-old hunter mare the day following onset of clinical signs of acute colitis. At initial examination packed cell volume and serum total protein were 65 l/l and 62 g/l, respectively, and continuous intravenous fluid therapy had been maintained.
(a) What disease processes, other than colitis, are indicated by these results?
(b) How would you further investigate this case?
(c) Outline a suitable therapeutic regimen for this case.
(d) What is the prognosis for this case?

Table 1

		Normal range
Blood biochemistry		
Sodium	125	134–143 mmol/l
Potassium	6.3	3.3–5.3 mmol/l
Chloride	91	89–106 mmol/l
Calcium	2.3	2.9–3.9 mmol/l
Phosphate	0.37	0.5–1.6 mmol/l
Urea	30.1	3.5–8.0 mmol/l
Creatinine	1328	90–180 μmol/l
Alkaline phosphatase	321	50–250 mmol/l
Glucose	3.9	3.5–5.9 mmol/l
Total protein	46	46–70 g/l
Albumin	22	17–37 g/l
Globulin	24	21–41 g/l
Haematology		
Red blood cells	8.11	$6.5–12.5 \times 10^2$/l
Packed cell volume	0.396	0.35–0.45 l/l
Haemoglobin	14.2	11.0–16.0 g/dl
Mean cell volume	49	31.0–41.0 fl
White blood cells	3.42	$4.0–10.0 \times 10^9$/l
Neutrophil	0.97	$1.4–5.8 \times 10^9$/l
Lymphocyte	2.05	$1.4–4.7 \times 10^9$/l
Monocyte	0.2	$0–0.2 \times 10^9$/l

96 A racehorse received an injury during a race, resulting in a cut to the skin on the plantar aspect of the metatarsus. This has subsequently swollen and refuses to heal (*Figure 78*). A discharge is present.
(a) What structures may be involved in the injury? How would you determine this?
(b) Why is healing delayed?
(c) What is your recommended treatment?

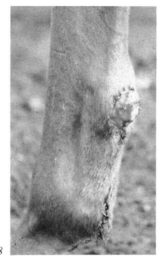

Figure 78

97 What are the palpable features (per rectum) of the reproductive tract of a pregnant mare at (a) 21 days, (b) 32 days, (c) 60 days, (d) 90 days, (e) 150 days and (f) 8 months?
Explain why each structure feels as it does.

98 A 6-year-old gelding, grazing with others, has been found with a fracture of the incisor quadrant of the left hemimandible (*Figure 79*). Can you suggest a simple method to restore the normal alignment of the teeth and to maintain fixation?

Figure 79

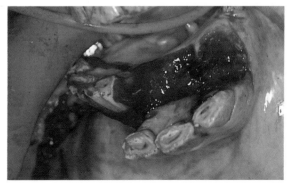

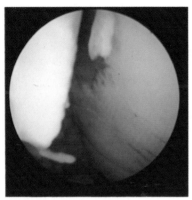

Figure 80

99 *Figure 80* demonstrates a displaced slab fracture of the third carpal bone, viewed from the dorsolateral aspect of the middle carpal joint.
(a) How may reduction of this fracture be aided and what is the treatment of choice?
(b) What is the most common site of such fractures?
(c) What other pathology is visible in this joint?

100 An owner asks whether additional fat (oil) should be fed.
(a) What possible major benefits of feeding additional fat to a horse could there be?
(b) Are these likely to apply to racehorses?
(c) Could feeding excess be harmful?
(d) What type of fat/oil should be fed?

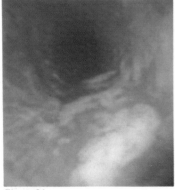

Figure 81

101 A pony is presented with acute onset dysphagia after known access to sugar beet pulp. Endoscopy has been performed because frequent coughing has been associated with the dysphagia; the state of the trachea is shown in *Figure 81*. What significance would you attach to this finding and what action should be taken?

Figure 82

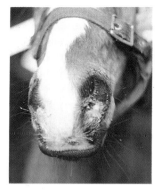

102 Five out of a group of 20 yearling Thoroughbreds on a stud farm have developed a respiratory disease characterised by anorexia, pyrexia (rectal temperature up to 40.5°C), coughing, purulent nasal discharge (*Figure 82*) and enlargement of the submandibular lymph nodes. A few of the affected horses have been dysphagic, and many of them have been standing with the neck and head outstretched. The first yearling became ill 10 days ago; the enlarged submandibular lymph nodes in this animal have burst, draining thick, creamy pus. In two of the other horses the nodes have started to fluctuate.
(a) What is the diagnosis?
(b) How would you treat the affected animals?
(c) What steps can be taken to limit the spread of the disease to the other yearlings?

103 A stallion has been led out to cover a mare and is observed to have a scab-encrusted lesion on the penis near the reflection of the prepuce (*Figure 83*).
(a) What is the most likely disease and what is the cause?
(b) Can it be transmitted to mares?
(c) Does it cause infertility?

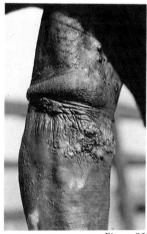

Figure 83

Figure 84

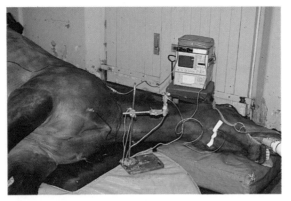

104 (a) What monitoring aids are illustrated in *Figure 84*?
(b) In your opinion which is the most important and why?

105 The lesion shown in *Figure 85* appeared slowly over a period of 2 weeks. The owner had blamed an ill-fitting saddle.
(a) What is the likely diagnosis?
(b) What public health aspects may be associated with it?
(c) What other diagnostic tests might you employ?
(d) What treatment regimen should be employed?

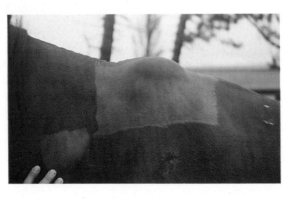

Figure 85

106 The 6-year-old mare in *Figure 86* has been showing
clinical signs for 6 weeks.
(a) What structure is affected?
(b) What further investigations are indicated?
(c) How will these aid in giving a prognosis?

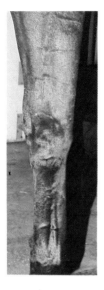

Figure 86

107 What factors are involved in the production and diagnosis of rectal tears
in horses?

108 A Shetland pony brood mare was
permanently stabled. In the month of June
she developed severe pruritus of the
tailhead, illustrated in *Figure 87*.
(a) What is this condition?
(b) What is the pathogenesis of the clinical
signs?
(c) How would you confirm the diagnosis?
(d) How would you manage this case?

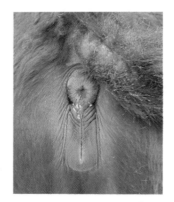

Figure 87

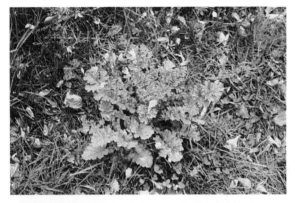

Figure 88A

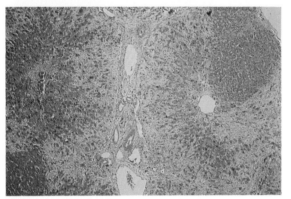

Figure 88B (reproduced with permission from *In Practice, Journal of Veterinary Postgraduate Clinical Study*)

109 Weight loss has been noticed in two of the four horses kept at a pasture containing many plants of the species shown in *Figure 88A*.
(a) Identify the plant and name its toxic principles.
(b) The histological section in *Figure 88B* is from a liver biopsy from one of the affected horses. Describe the pathological changes (stain: Masson's trichrome; magnification: × 40).
(c) What is the mechanism of action of the toxin?
(d) What is the best single screening test to detect the subclinical liver damage which might have occurred in the two apparently normal horses?

110 A 4-year-old pony gelding was presented for investigation of marked weight loss over the preceding month. The animal had a normal appetite and a moderately increased thirst. The only finding on physical examination was that the animal was in very poor body condition. Urine from the pony had a normal specific gravity and contained 2% glucose. The results of haematological, blood biochemical analyses are given in *Table 2*.
(a) What is the probable diagnosis?
(b) What is the likely cause of the condition?
(c) How would you further investigate this case?

Table 2

		Normal range
Blood biochemistry		
Sodium	136	134–143 mmol/l
Potassium	3.6	3.3–5.3 mmol/l
Chloride	92	89–106 mmol/l
Calcium	2.9	2.9–3.9 mmol/l
Phosphate	0.64	0.5–1.6 mmol/l
Urea	4.6	3.5–8.0 mmol/l
Creatinine	135	90–180 µmol/l
Alkaline phosphatase	430	50–250 mmol/l
Gamma glutamyl transferase	87	<40 iu/l
Glucose	10.6	3.5–5.9 mmol/l
Total protein	68	46–70 g/l
Albumin	32	17–37 g/l
Globulin	36	21–41 g/l
Haematology		
Red blood cells	6.8	$6.5–12.5 \times 10^2$/l
Packed cell volume	0.370	0.35–0.45 l/l
Haemoglobin	13.7	11.0–16.0 g/dl
Mean cell volume	36	31.0–41.0 fl
White blood cells	7.23	$4.0–10.0 \times 10^9$/l
Neutrophil	4.34	$1.4–5.8 \times 10^9$/l
Lymphocyte	2.53	$1.4–4.7 \times 10^9$/l
Monocyte	0.20	$0–0.2 \times 10^9$/l
Eosinophil	0.16	

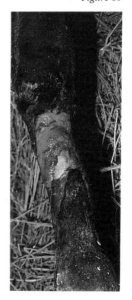

Figure 89

111 The injury illustrated in *Figure 89* occurred 3 weeks previously. In some areas healing by granulation tissue is progressing satisfactorily but an area of exposed bone persists.
(a) What is the probable problem?
(b) How could it be treated?
(c) Would the area then granulate over?

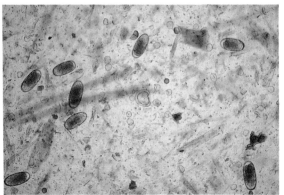

Figure 90

112 (a) What is the significance of the structures shown on the faecal smear illustrated in *Figure 90*?
(b) What should be the next course of investigation?
(c) Should the owner take any precautions?

113 A normal scrotal testicle (left) and an incomplete abdominally retained testicle (right) are illustrated in *Figure 91*.
(a) What structures are marked?
(b) How may cryptorchidism be classified in the horse?
(c) How is it possible to confirm the presence of testicular tissue in an apparently castrated horse?

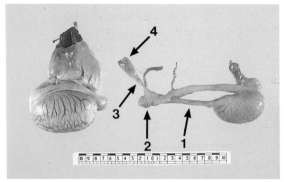

Figure 91 (courtesy of Dr J.S.E. David, University of Bristol)

114 A 10-year-old pony mare has been affected by chronic diarrhoea for 7 months. The pony has remained bright and alert, although she has lost some weight, and the owners have been able to continue to work her throughout the course of her illness. Faecal consistency has been variable, ranging from soft ('cowpat') to watery. The pony is stabled during the winter, and kept at pasture during the summer. She has been well managed, and regularly wormed at 6-week intervals since purchase at 3 years of age. Repeated clinical and laboratory examinations (haematology, serum biochemistry profiles, parasitological, bacteriological and cytological examination of faeces) have been unremarkable. Likewise, peritoneal fluid analysis, oral glucose tolerance tests and a rectal biopsy have revealed no abnormalities.
(a) What is the likely cause of the diarrhoea in this animal?
(b) Are there any other diagnostic tests that may be of help?
(c) What treatments would you advise?

115 (a) What are the hepatic lesions shown in *Figure 92*?
(b) Are the lesions of pathogenic significance?
(c) Are the lesions of zoonotic significance?

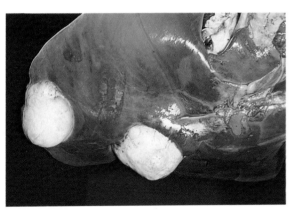

Figure 92

116 Seven horses in a large livery yard have developed a mild respiratory disease characterised by a serous or mucoid nasal discharge, coughing, mild fever and inappetence. The submandibular lymph nodes have shown slight enlargement in affected animals. All horses in the yard are stabled on straw and are fed hay. They have all been vaccinated against equine influenza within the past 12 months.
(a) What is the likely diagnosis?
(b) How would you treat the affected animals?

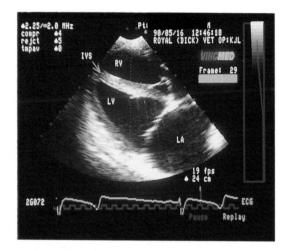

Figure 93. Right ventricle (RV); left ventricle (LV); interventricular septum (IVS); left atrium (LA).

117 A 3-year-old pony presented with a grade 5/6 pansystolic murmur over the right hemithorax. The point of maximum intensity of the murmur was over the tricuspid valve region, but it could also be heard ventrally and cranially along the sternal border. A precordial thrill was present. The second heart sound was louder than normal.
(a) What is the most likely cause of this murmur?
(b) What information can be gained from the echocardiogram (*Figure 93*) to indicate the severity of the condition?
(c) Which area of the heart would you image in order to confirm your diagnosis?
(d) What is the likely prognosis in this case?

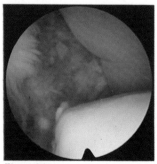

Figure 94

118 *Figure 94* demonstrates a chip fracture from the dorsodistal articular margin of the radial carpal bone.
(a) Does this arthroscopic appearance suggest that the fracture is acute or chronic?
(b) Which radiographic views are most useful in demonstrating the presence of such chip fractures?

119 (a) What is the plant in *Figure 95* and is it important?
(b) What clinical condition may it cause?
(c) How are horses affected most often?

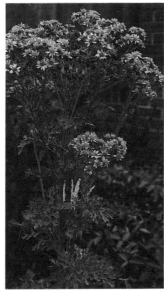

Figure 95

120 A hard swelling which is slightly bilobed and lies symmetrically across the nasal midline of this horse has developed over 3 weeks (*Figure 96*). What is the significance of the lesion and how would you confirm your diagnosis?

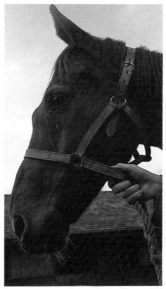

Figure 96

59

Figure 97

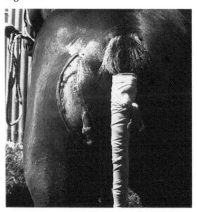

121 A fresh vertical skin wound on a horse's buttock, illustrated in *Figure 97*, occurred when the horse backed rapidly off a horse transporter into a protruding sheet of iron.
(a) Can it be repaired and if so, describe how you would do it?
(b) Will the repair be successful?
(c) Will there be any loss of function?

122 A 4-hour-old, 340-day gestational age Arabian filly is presented with a history of weakness since birth. The birth process was observed to be normal, and the mare has had three normal foals previously. On physical examination, the mucous membranes are cyanotic, and the respiratory rate is 40 breaths/min. Thoracic auscultation reveals harsh lung sounds, with no wheezes or crackles; no unusual heart murmurs are noted. On arterial blood gas analysis, Po_2 is 20 mmHg, Pco_2 is 45 mmHg, and pH 7.2.
(a) What are the most likely differential diagnoses?
(b) What is your diagnostic plan?

123 A 3-year-old Thoroughbred mare was presented with a 3-month history of weight loss, inappetence, lethargy, polydipsia and polyuria. Rectal examination revealed an enlarged spleen, which had a 'lumpy' surface texture. The heart rate was elevated (50 beats/min) and a pansystolic murmur was audible over the left side. The results of some of the laboratory estimations are shown.

	Case	Normal
PCV (l/l)	21	36–52
RBC × 10^{12}/l	4.75	7.5–11.0
Haemoglobin (g/dl)	7.6	14–19
WBC × 10^9/l	13.6	5–9
Fibrinogen (g/l)	8.4	2–4
Urea (mmol/l)	7.3	3.2–5.2
Creatinine (μmol/l)	134	128–188
Calcium (mmol/l)	3.9	2.8–3.1
Urine sp. gr.	1.018	1.020–1.050

(cont.)

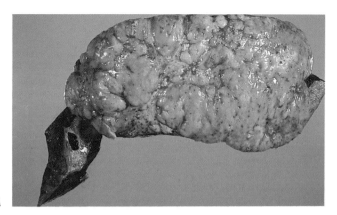

Figure 98A

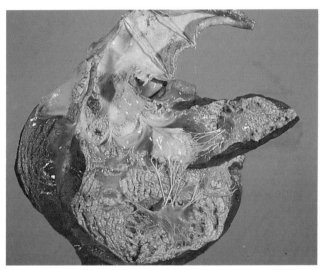

Figure 98B

123 (*cont.*) The horse was destroyed on humanitarian grounds. Post-mortem examination revealed an enlarged spleen which was mostly replaced by firm, nodular, pale tissue (*Figure 98A*). Calcification of the endocardium of all four heart chambers, the heart valves and lining of the aorta was also found (*Figure 98B*).
(a) What are the relevant clinicopathological findings?
(b) What is the likely diagnosis, and how does this explain the clinical signs?

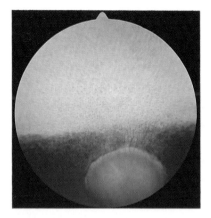

Figure 99

124 (a) Is the retina shown in *Figure 99* (from a 6-year-old hunter) normal?
(b) What are the distinguishing ophthalmoscopic features?

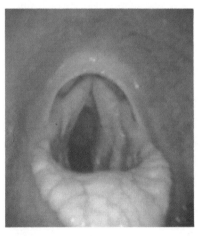

125 *Figure 100* shows the endoscopic view of the larynx of a 2-year-old Thoroughbred filly reported to produce abnormal respiratory noises at exercise. What is your diagnosis and what other signs might the filly have shown?

Figure 100

126 The 18-year-old New Forest pony mare (shown in *Figure 101*) was recently involved in an accident, when the trailer in which it was travelling overturned on a motorway. After this, it was severely lame on the right hindlimb.
(a) What is the differential diagnosis?
(b) What investigation is indicated?
(c) How will this affect the advice to the owner?

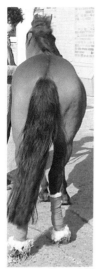

Figure 101

127 A 6-year-old Shetland pony is presented with dullness, abdominal pain, diarrhoea and ventral oedema in late pregnancy. The oral mucosa is shown in *Figure 102*.
(a) What abnormalities are visible?
(b) What is the most likely diagnosis?
(c) How would you confirm the diagnosis?
(d) How would you treat this case?
(e) Which laboratory tests could be used to monitor progress?

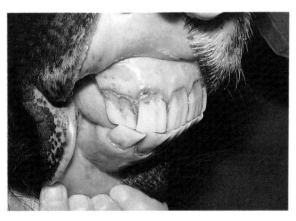

Figure 102

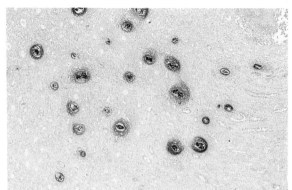

Figure 103

128 *Figure 103* shows a photomicrograph of a section of kidney from a 4-year-old Thoroughbred gelding which had a 6-month history of polyuria, polydipsia and a moderate loss of body weight (stain: von Kossa; magnification: × 99).
(a) What is the diagnosis?
(b) What other pathological features are likely to be present in this case?

129 At what stage of pregnancy can twin conception be first detected by:
(a) Ultrasonography.
(b) Palpation.

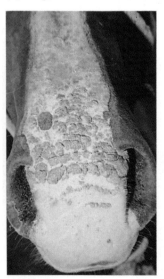

130 Several horses grazing in a paddock are presented with loss of hair from the face, body and legs. Close examination shows exudation and matting of the hair with excessive scab formation (*Figure 104*). There appears to be little to no pruritus. Lesions are not restricted to white areas.
(a) What is your diagnosis and what is a common name for this condition?
(b) What specimens are needed to confirm this?
(c) Does the organism require any special cultural conditions?
(d) Name a treatment which could be effectively used.

Figure 104

131 The frontal sinus of this horse has been entered using a skin flap and resection of a piece of frontal bone (*Figure 105*).
(a) What are the surgical landmarks for access to the frontal and maxillary sinuses in the horse?
(b) What considerations should be addressed when making a surgical approach to the paranasal sinuses in the horse?
(c) What are the common complications of sinus surgery in the horse and how are they managed?

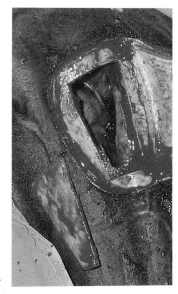

Figure 105

132 A myelogram is shown (*Figure 106*) of a 250-kg foal, obtained with the neck in flexion. At which intervertebral site(s) is there a lesion(s)?

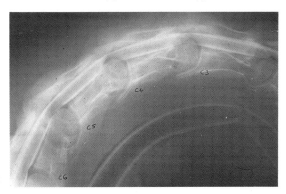

Figure 106

133 What is the value of determining plasma progesterone concentrations in the blood of pregnant mares?

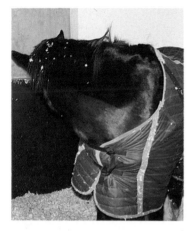

Figure 107

134 Two hours after exercise this 7-year-old pony gelding (*Figure 107*) showed moderate colic signs. Bowel sounds were increased, particularly during episodes of pain. Between bouts of pain the pulse was 35/min. Mucous membranes were normal. Per rectum no abnormalities were detected. There was no gastric reflux.
(a) What is your diagnosis?
(b) How would you treat this case?
(c) What medication would you avoid?
(d) How would you proceed?

135 A fresh horizontal wound (*Figure 108)* of the thigh region is presented for treatment.
(a) Is suturing likely to be successful?
(b) If the wound is sutured when are complications likely to occur?
(c) What would be the best treatment if wound breakdown occurred?
(d) What is your initial treatment of choice?

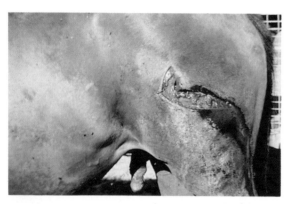

Figure 108

136 A 3-year-old Thoroughbred racehorse became acutely ill 1 h after returning home from a race meeting. The horse was depressed, and had projectile, watery, foul-smelling diarrhoea. Conjunctival and oral mucous membranes were congested; capillary refill time was prolonged (4.5 s). The heart rate was elevated (86 beats/min), and there was tachypnoea (respiratory rate 28/min). Rectal temperature was elevated (39.0°C), but the extremities felt cold to the touch. Rectal examination revealed no abnormalities other than the presence of watery rectal contents.

Intensive intravenous therapy with fluids and electrolytes was initiated, but the horse died 6 h later. The section shown in *Figure 109* (haematoxylin and eosin stain) was obtained from the large colon.
(a) Describe the histological changes.
(b) What gross post-mortem findings would be consistent with the pathological changes illustrated?
(c) What is the differential diagnosis?
(d) How should the diagnosis be established?

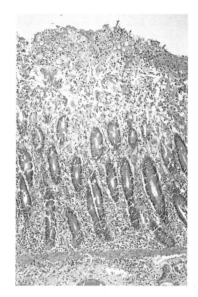

Figure 109

Figure 110

137 (a) What information can be gained from the endoscopic view, illustrated in *Figure 110*, of the pharynx of a young horse?
(b) Is the animal in any immediate danger?
(c) How do you explain the difference between the two sides?

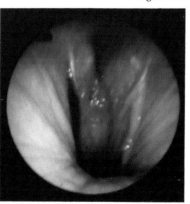

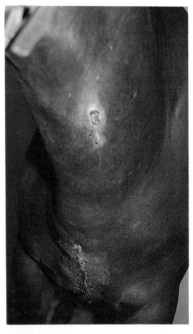

Figure 111

138 The horse shown in *Figure 111* developed these discharging sinuses on its neck 10 days after general anaesthesia. A stormy induction had occurred.

(a) What drug or drugs were probably used to induce anaesthesia in this animal?

(b) How would you have treated this accident: immediately after induction of the original anaesthetic, or approximately 10 days after the anaesthetic?

(c) How can such accidents be avoided?

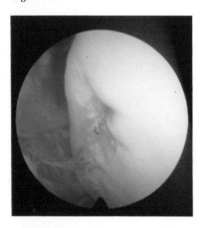

Figure 112

139 A 3-year-old Thoroughbred racehorse had a history of persistent forelimb lameness which was relieved by local analgesia of the middle carpal joint. Arthroscopic examination revealed this defect in the radial facet of the third carpal bone (*Figure 112*).

(a) What is this lesion?

(b) Which radiographic projection is most useful in identifying such lesions?

(c) What extra-articular structure is found overlying this area?

140 A 3-year-old colt has returned home having been stabled elsewhere for 3 days at a far-distant race meeting. This colt originally manifested a mild fever, anorexia and dullness. Initially, auscultation suggested ileus, but diarrhoea developed within the succeeding 24 h. A leucopenia with degenerative left shift has been noted on a sample submitted for clinical pathology examination. These factors are believed to be associated with 'colitis'. What additional laboratory assessments and replacement fluids would be of value in the management of this case?

141 A 7-year-old show jumper gelding presented with a variable degree of lameness of several weeks' duration. Lameness was not improved by perineural analgesia of the palmar (abaxial sesamoid) nerves but was alleviated by analgesia of the palmar (mid cannon) and palmar metacarpal nerves. Radiographs of the metacarpophalangeal joint were obtained.
(a) What views would you obtain?
(b) Describe the radiographic features shown in *Figure 113*.
(c) How would you determine the significance of the separate body?
(d) What is its differential diagnosis?
(e) What treatment would you recommend?
(f) What is your prognosis?

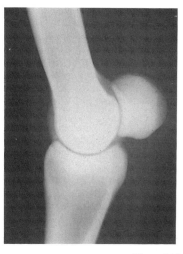

Figure 113

142 You are consulted by the worried owner of a mare that has not foaled 350 days after service. How would you treat this problem?

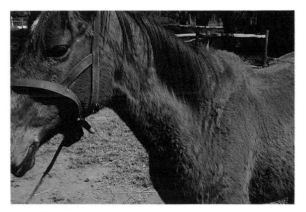

Figure 114

143 The picture of this horse (*Figure 114*) was obtained in the middle of summer.
(a) What is your suspected diagnosis and why?
(b) What other clinical signs may occur with this condition?
(c) Would the disorder be expected to improve?
(d) Can the signs be attributed to a heavy worm burden?

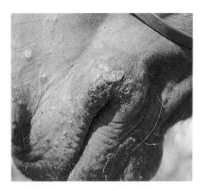

Figure 115

144 A young horse in a subtropical country has recently been returned from a horse handler where it has been taught to lead. A painful area is located on the right commissure of the mouth (*Figure 115*). When cleaned, it is found to contain a granular-type lumpy purulent material. The horse is obviously irritated and constantly rubs at the lesion.
(a) What is the condition due to?
(b) What is your differential diagnosis?
(c) What treatment would you recommend?

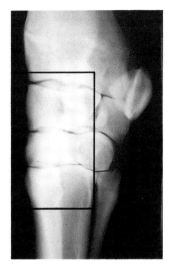

Figure 116A

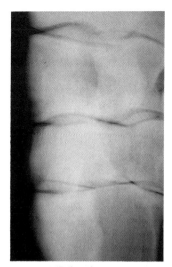

Figure 116B (inset)

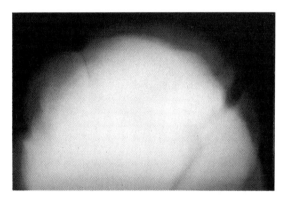

Figure 116C

145 A 4-year-old Thoroughbred racehorse presented with right forelimb lameness of 10 days' duration. There was slight distension of the middle carpal joint capsule and lameness was alleviated by intra-articular analgesia of the joint.
(a) What radiographic views would you obtain?
(b) What projections are shown in *Figures 116A and C*?
(c) Describe the radiographic features in *Figures 116A–C*.
(d) What is your diagnosis, treatment and prognosis?

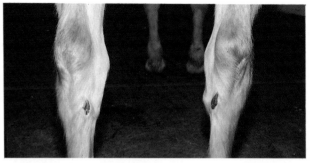

Figure 117

146 The 9-year-old pony mare, whose limbs are shown in *Figure 117*, was lame on its left forelimb.
(a) What clinical observation(s) do you make and to what condition may it be related?
(b) Is this likely to be causing a clinical problem?

147 The pressure traces shown in *Figure 118* were taken with a dual sensor micromanometer-tipped catheter placed in the left atrium and left ventricle. A simultaneous lead Y ECG is also shown. The pressures are measured in mmHg, the scale is shown on the left; paper speed 25 mm/s.
(a) Name six abnormalities.
(b) What is the most likely explanation of these findings?
(c) What are the likely presenting signs in this case?

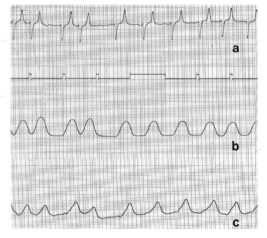

Figure 118. (a) Lead Y; (b) left ventricular heart pressure (mm Hg); (c) left atrial pressure (mm Hg); paper speed, 25 mm/sec.

148 (a) Which surgical approach is used for routine exploration of the equine abdomen?
- Ventral midline.
- Paramedian.
- Flank.
- Inguinal.

(b) Describe the location of the ventral midline incision relative to the umbilicus.

(c) What is the importance of an incision precisely dividing the linea alba?

(d) Why is it recommended to start every exploration of the abdomen with exteriorisation of the caecum?

(e) Closure of the ventral midline laparotomy incision can be performed in three or four layers. Which are the layers concerned and which suture materials would you use for each of them and why?

149 (a) What clinical signs can you detect in *Figure 119*?
(b) Can these signs be attributed to a fall on the race track?
(c) What other causes for this might be identifiable?
(d) What is the prognosis for the horse?

Figure 119

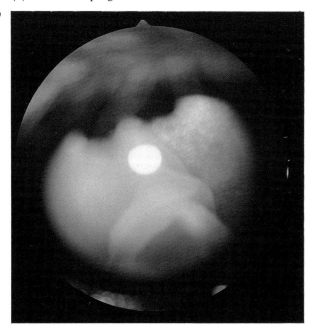

150 What treatment would you suggest to prevent pregnancy after misalliance in a mare?

151 The traditional trephine and repulsion of a maxillary cheek tooth is demonstrated in *Figure 120*.
(a) What other surgical approaches may be used for removal of dental tissue in the horse?
(b) What are the relative merits of these techniques?
(c) What are the common complications of equine dental surgery?

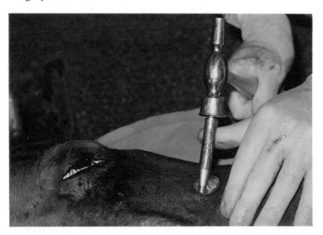

Figure 120

152 In what circumstance does fetal mummification occur?

153 A severe wound to the carpus in a breeding mare is presented for treatment 12 h after a storm (*Figure 121*). There is no involvement of the carpal joints.
(a) Would you attempt to suture this wound?
(b) How would you manage the first week's treatment?
(c) Would you expect this wound to heal with a high degree of normal function, if properly treated?

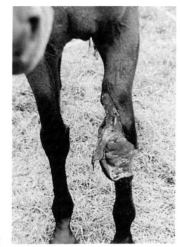

Figure 121

154 Various swabs are used in the isolation and identification of bacterial and viral infections in horses. Examples of some swab types appear in *Figure 122*. Which swab would be appropriate for:
(a) Investigation of venereal disease in a stallion.
(b) Preparation of a cervico-endometrial smear.
(c) Virus isolation in a suspected outbreak of respiratory disease involving EHV1.
(d) Taking a sample of the flora of the clitoral sinus and fossa.
(e) Attempting to confirm a suspected case of *Streptococcus equi* infection.

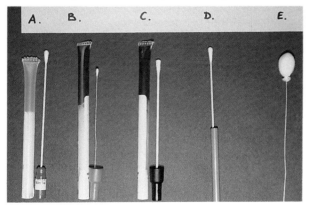

Figure 122

155 The surgical colic patient remains hospitalised 1–2 weeks depending on the occurrence of complications in the postoperative period.
(a) Which perioperative antibiotics can be used routinely and for how long? Why should the period of antibiotic administration be kept to a minimum?
(b) When is the patient reintroduced to water and food? Which food materials can be used in the early feeding programme?
Once the animal is discharged from the hospital, adequate advice concerning further convalescence will be sought.
(c) When can the skin sutures be removed?
(d) Will the horse have to be box rested or is paddock rest acceptable? When can the animal resume normal exercise? Is any form of earlier light exercise possible? Why is restriction of exercise necessary?
(e) What nutritional guidelines can be given?

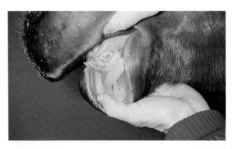

Figure 123A

156 The horse shown in *Figures 123A* and *B* had been treated for a mild upper respiratory tract infection some 4 weeks previously.
(a) Name four clinical signs which are present.
(b) What is your differential diagnosis?
(c) What conditions may precede the appearance of these signs and help in the establishment of a definitive diagnosis?
(d) Will a blood sample reveal any pathognomonic features?

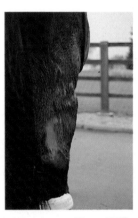

Figure 123B

157 You are asked to examine for soundness a 4-year-old hunter and you find an abnormality of the right eye (*Figure 124*).
(a) What is your diagnosis?
(b) What other features do you notice?
(c) What is your advice?

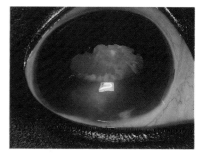

Figure 124

158 An 8-year-old Thoroughbred racehorse in a large National Hunt yard has been showing unusually poor form and reduced exercise tolerance over a 3-month period. The trainer has noticed that the horse has been coughing at the start of exercise, but not at any other time. There is no nasal discharge or pyrexia, and the horse seems well in all other respects. Routine haematological and serum biochemical profiles have been consistently normal. Clinical examinations at rest have been unremarkable, and there is no obvious adventitious respiratory noise at exercise. You suspect low grade lower airway disease.
(a) What is the likely diagnosis?
(b) What diagnostic procedures could you utilise to confirm the presence of lower airway disease?

159 The arthroscopic photograph in *Figure 125* is a view of the distal aspect of the trochlear ridges and intertrochlear groove of the femur and associated synovial membranes in a National Hunt horse with a history of repeated exercise-induced femoropatellar joint distension and lameness. No osteochondral pathology was identified radiographically or at arthroscopy.
(a) What is your tentative diagnosis?
(b) What other diagnostic tests might be performed?

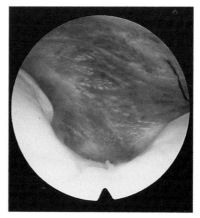

Figure 125

160 An 8-year-old Thoroughbred gelding finished the cross country phase of a three-day event lame on the right hindlimb. One gram of phenylbutazone, administered with permission of the Ground Jury, rendered the horse sufficiently sound to compete on the final day, but the following day lameness deteriorated, associated with distension of the femoropatellar joint capsule. Radiographs of the stifle were obtained.
(a) Describe the radiographic findings shown in *Figure 126*.
(b) What additional radiographic views would you obtain and why?
(c) What is the likely aetiology of the separate osseous body?
(d) What is your treatment and prognosis?

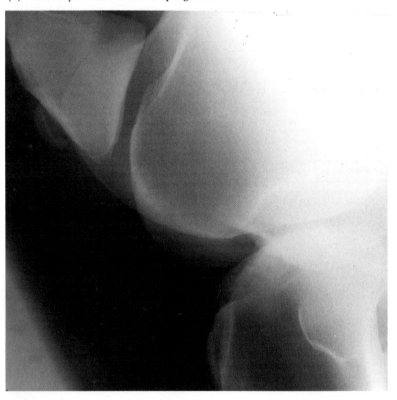

Figure 126

161 The following laboratory results were obtained from a suspected case of grass sickness of 2 days' duration:

Test	Case	Normal
PCV (l/l)	0.48	0.24–0.40
Total serum protein (g/l)	85	58–75
Blood urea (mmol/l)	15	2.5–8.3
Plasma cortisol	942	60–170
Serum alkaline phosphatase (iu/l)	250	84–180

(a) How would you interpret the laboratory findings?
(b) Which other laboratory tests might have been useful in supporting the ante-mortem diagnosis?

162 A yearling is being prepared for sale when the owner calls you to examine some warts around the horse's eye (*Figure 127*). He wishes to sell the yearling in 3 weeks.
(a) What is the condition and is it infectious?
(b) How would you treat this particular horse?
(c) Why?
(d) If the warts were around the nose, would they require treatment?

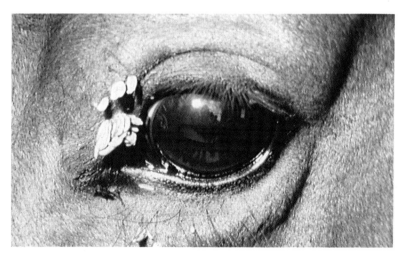

Figure 127

Figure 128

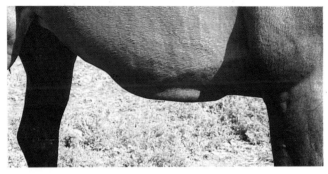

163 List the common diagnostic possibilities for the clinical sign shown in *Figure 128*.

164 A 7-year-old point-to-point horse pulled up acutely lame during a training gallop. A deep puncture wound was identified on the palmar aspect of the pastern. Synovial fluid was not detected. The horse was treated with broad-spectrum sytemic antimicrobial drugs and a non-steroidal anti-inflammatory drug. The horse made progressive improvement but then had a relapse associated with distension of the flexor tendon sheath. The horse showed moderate lameness at the walk. An ultrasonographic examination of the soft tissues on the palmar aspect of the pastern was performed (*Figure 129*).
(a) What structures can you identify?
(b) Are there any abnormalities?
(c) What other diagnostic tests would you perform?
(d) How would you treat the horse?
(e) What is your prognosis?

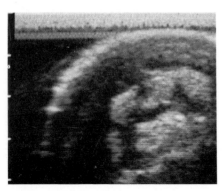

Figure 129

Figure 130

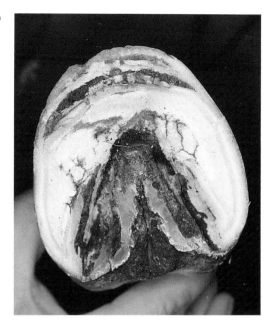

165 A 3-month-old half-bred colt presented for flexural deformity of a distal interphalangeal joint.
(a) What problem is illustrated in *Figure 130*?
(b) Would a radiograph of the foot be helpful?
(c) How might the secondary problem affect the treatment of this case?

166 An owner asks how he can 'glycogen load' his horse.
(a) Is it possible to increase a horse's glycogen stores?
(b) Is glycogen loading likely to be of any benefit?
(c) What possible detrimental effects of glycogen loading could there be?

167 What is the 'holding injection' which is given to mares and in what circumstances would you consider its use?

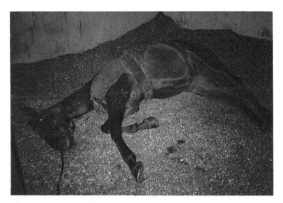

Figure 131

168 An 8-year-old hunter (*Figure 131*) was presented with signs of mild abdominal pain of 6 h duration. Pulse was 35/min and had normal character, mucous membranes were slightly injected and temperature and respiration normal. Capillary refill time was 1 s. Bowel sounds were depressed but occasionally loud borborygmi, which appeared to be associated with pain, could be auscultated in the left flank. There was no gastric reflux and faecal production was scanty. Per rectum the pelvic flexure was distended with a firm mass of ingesta which could be palpated in the pelvic canal.
(a) What is your diagnosis?
(b) How would you treat the case?
(c) Do you have any follow-up management advice?

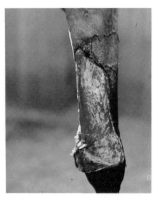

169 *Figure 132* shows a degloving injury to the forearm involving the skin and carpus. It occurred only 1 h ago.
(a) What is the best method of repair?
(b) Would you expect good healing from your treatment?

Figure 132

170 The sign shown in *Figure 133* had occurred several times in a circus horse over a 4-week period and one episode had been severe.
(a) Would it be useful to carry out a full blood profile with analysis of clotting function?
(b) What further diagnostic steps would be advisable?

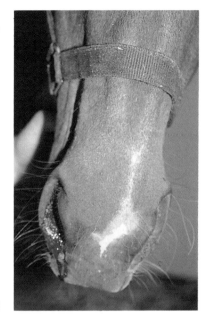

Figure 133

171 A 9-year-old Thoroughbred gelding (body weight 500 kg) suffered a fracture of the middle phalanx of the right forelimb, which was repaired surgically. The horse was hospitalised postoperatively, and treated with flunixin meglumine (500 mg two to three times a day as felt necessary) and procaine penicillin G (7.5 MU twice a day). Fourteen days after the surgery the horse developed fever, depression, anorexia, colic, and shortly thereafter profuse watery diarrhoea with severe dehydration. He was treated with intravenous fluids, systemic antibiotics (trimethoprim–sulphadiazine), analgesics, and flunixin meglumine, but 36 h later developed acute laminitis, and was destroyed on humanitarian grounds. Post-mortem examination revealed severe ulceration and inflammation confined to the right dorsal colon. What is the likely cause of this condition?

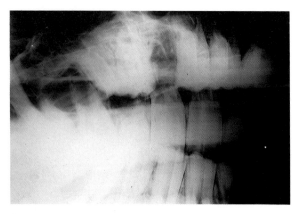

Figure 134

172 An adult horse was treated for secondary dental sinusitis by trephination and repulsion of the fourth upper cheek tooth. One month later the horse continued to have a unilateral, foul-smelling nasal discharge. The radiograph illustrated in *Figure 134* was obtained under general anaesthesia.
(a) What radiographic view has been used?
(b) What radiographic features can be seen?
(c) What is the aetiology of the continued nasal discharge?

173 The following arterial blood gas values were obtained from a foal spontaneously ventilating under general anaesthesia (halothane in oxygen):

	Case	*Normal*
pH	7.276	7.35–7.45
Pco_2	72.1 mmHg	35–45 mmHg
Po_2	269.8 mmHg	>100 mmHg

(a) What abnormality is present?
(b) How would you treat it?

174 A 5-year-old pony gelding was found with a profuse nasal discharge containing food material and saliva following feeding. It appeared to be retching occasionally.
(a) What is the most likely diagnosis and what other diagnostic possibilities should you take into account?
(b) How would you treat this?
(c) What follow-up measures would you advise?

Figure 135

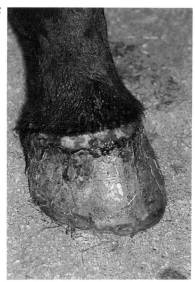

175 A 5-year-old mare has been losing weight for 3 months. Her appetite has been variable, and the faeces have been loose intermittently. Recently she has developed ventral oedema, and severe ulcerative coronitis (*Figure 135*) and stomatitis, with alopecia and hyperkeratosis over the muzzle and face. There has also been intense pruritus, which has not improved with corticosteroid therapy. Serum biochemistry has shown hypoalbuminaemia (albumin 16.5 g/l) and an oral glucose tolerance test revealed minimal glucose absorption.
(a) What is the likely diagnosis, and how can you confirm this?
(b) What is its aetiology and treatment?

176 A 4-year-old gelding with a history of ill thrift and poor performance is presented to you. Clinical examination of the horse has been unremarkable. The owners have given anthelmintic preparations to the horse at irregular intervals. Faecal examination has not demonstrated the presence of worm eggs, and yet you remain concerned at the possibility of otherwise inapparent parasitism. Is there another clinical pathology aid to diagnosis that might assist you in this case?

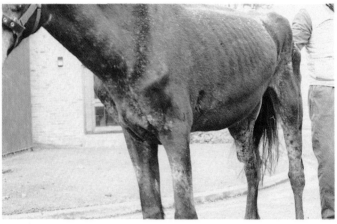

Figure 136

177 (a) What identifiable clinical features are apparent in *Figure 136*?
(b) What might be responsible for these?
(c) Can the condition be treated?

178 Vital signs were normal in the Thoroughbred foal shown in *Figure 137* which presented with an audible inspiratory dyspnoea.
(a) How do you explain the dyspnoea?
(b) What is the likely differential diagnosis?
(c) What further diagnostic steps may be used to confirm the diagnosis?

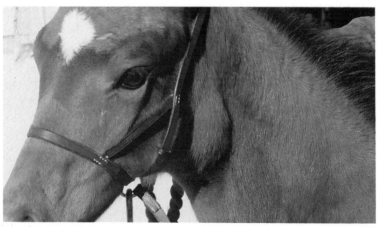

Figure 137

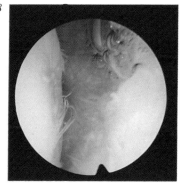

Figure 138

179 The articular opening of a subchondral bone cyst in the medial femoral condyle is shown in *Figure 138*.
(a) What is the commonest site of subchondral bone cysts (osseous cyst-like lesions)?
(b) How may the clinical significance of such lesions be determined?
(c) What are the two suggested surgical treatments?
(d) What further information is necessary before undertaking surgical treatment?

180 A carriage horse driver is concerned by the presence of a large fly around the horses' head and legs, causing them to be restless. He also notices the presence of small white to yellowish eggs on the hairs of the legs and chest (*Figure 139*).
(a) What could the fly be?
(b) What treatment could you recommend?
(c) What makes the eggs hatch?
(d) How do the larvae gain entry to the horse?

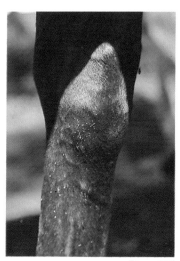

Figure 139

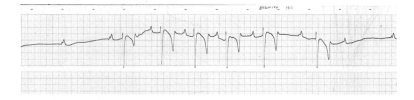

Figure 140. Lead Y; paper speed, 25 mm/sec.

181 The lead 'Y' ECG shown in *Figure 140* was obtained from an 8-year-old showjumper immediately after light trotting exercise.
(a) What does the ECG show?
(b) How would you investigate this further?
(c) Is this condition likely to affect the horse's performance?

182 An 8-year-old Thoroughbred chaser gelding is presented at a referral hospital with a 20-h history of continuous moderate-to-severe abdominal discomfort. The attending veterinary surgeon has administered the following drugs during his consecutive visits: 160 mg hyoscine-*N*-butylbromide and 20 g dipyrone (Buscopan compositum), 50 mg butorphanol (Torbugesic), 240 mg xylazine (Rompun) and 1 g flunixin meglumine (Finadyne).

On presentation the horse is depressed, sweating and in continuous pain, trying to go down. Heart rate is 42 beats/min, respiratory rate is 32/min and PCV is 34%. Bowel sounds are absent. On passage of a stomach tube there is reflux of gastric fluid. Rectal examination reveals the presence of numerous distended loops of small intestine and an inspissated left colon (*Figure 141*).

(a) What other diagnostic procedure should be undertaken?
(b) What action would you advise?
(c) Which parameters guide the choice of treatment?
(d) In view of the final diagnosis, why did the animal present with cardiovascular parameters within normal limits?

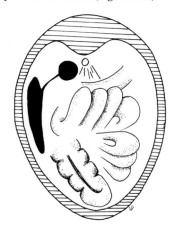

Figure 141. Rectal findings.

183 (a) What significant features can you identify in the inguinal region of this horse (*Figure 142A*)?
(b) Describe the lesions shown in *Figure 142B*.
(c) What other features would be found?
(d) What public health aspects should be considered?

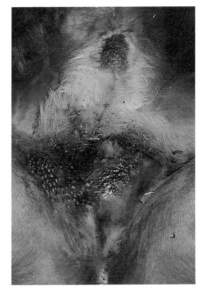

Figure 142A

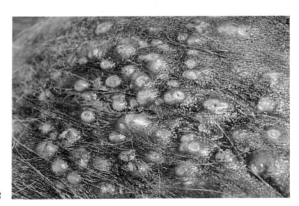

Figure 142B

184 (a) Why are 'membrane slip' and placentomes not palpable features of pregnancy in mares?
(b) What is the significance of feeling fremitus in the middle uterine artery?

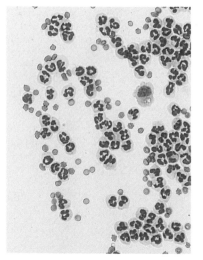

Figure 143A

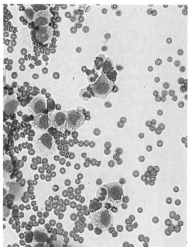

Figure 143B

185 The smears in *Figure 143* were prepared from synovial fluid taken from a tarsocrural joint of a Thoroughbred colt at 2 weeks of age (*Figure 143A*) and 4 weeks of age (*Figure 143B*).
(a) What is the differential diagnosis?
(b) What treatment is the animal likely to have received between 2 and 4 weeks of age?
(c) Has the problem been controlled?

186 The following laboratory results were obtained from a horse showing intermittent, mild colic and anorexia of 4 days' duration. General examination revealed no obvious abnormalities other than poor body condition.

Test	Case	Normal
Total protein (g/l)	90.4	58–75
Albumin (g/l)	21.2	23–35
Globulin (g/l)	69.2	30–58
Blood urea (mmol/l)	1.9	2.5–8.3
Aspartate aminotransferase (iu/l)	624	258–554
Glutamate dehydrogenase (iu/l)	481	1–12
Total bilirubin (μmol/l)	38	17–34

(a) How would you interpret the laboratory findings?
(b) What additional investigations should be undertaken?

187 A 9-year-old Thoroughbred gelding was admitted to a hospital with a history of colic for the last 3 days. Diagnosis of a large impaction of the left colon had been made, but this had failed to clear with standard treatment. The animal was given appropriate therapy and progress was assessed by repeated rectal examination during the next 48 h. On one of these examinations the clinician experienced a sudden feeling of release of pressure on the arm followed by abnormally easy palpation of viscera. On withdrawal he detected the presence of fresh blood on his rectal sleeve.

(a) What is the likely diagnosis?
(b) What is the most common location and direction of this injury?
(c) An immediate evaluation of the injury is necessary. What steps should be taken to facilitate this initial examination?
(d) What are the most important facts to determine during the initial evaluation? How are such injuries classified?
(e) What is the best course of action for each of the different gradations of the injury?

188 What neurological deficit is apparent in the horse illustrated in *Figure 144*? Can you speculate on the site of the lesion?

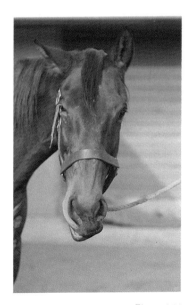

Figure 144

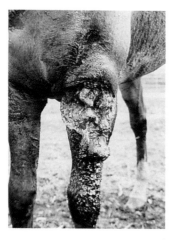

Figure 145

189 A racehorse has been injured during a storm and has a large avulsion wound on the forearm, with damage to skin and extensor muscles (*Figure 145*).
(a) How would you treat this wound?
(b) If the extensor muscles are severely torn, would the horse still be able to race without impairment?
(c) How long would you expect the wound to take to heal fully? Would you give graded exercise, or no exercise during the healing period?

190 What is the significance of:
(a) Lactation during mid to late pregnancy?
(b) Slight vaginal haemorrhage in mid to late pregnancy?

191 (a) Would the lesion illustrated in *Figure 146* be likely to affect the animal's metabolic status and what biochemical changes would be found?
(b) What other swellings may occur in this area?
(c) Would it be likely to cause respiratory embarrassment?

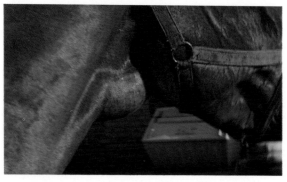

Figure 146

192 A 4-year-old Thoroughbred gelding has been showing progressive weight loss for 3 months. His appetite has been poor, and he has also demonstrated intermittent pyrexia and low grade abdominal pain. The prepuce has become oedematous (*Figure 147*). A haematological and serum biochemical profile have revealed no specific abnormalities other than hypoalbuminaemia (albumin 19.6 g/l).

An oral glucose tolerance test was performed by administering glucose at a dose rate of 1 g/kg as a 20% solution by stomach tube after an overnight fast. The results are shown below·

Time after administration of glucose (min)	Plasma glucose (mmol/l)
0 (pre-administration)	4.0
30	4.3
60	4.1
90	4.1
120	4.0
180	4.0

(a) Describe the expected absorption test results in a normal horse.
(b) How do you interpret these results?
(c) What types of diseases do you suspect?
(d) What is the prognosis?

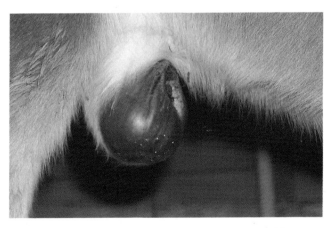

Figure 147

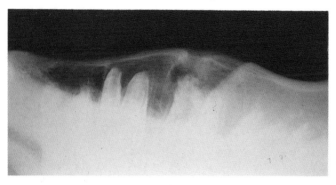

Figure 148

193 The radiograph shown in *Figure 148* was obtained from a horse presented with a unilateral mandibular swelling and an associated sinus tract discharging ventrally.
(a) From the presenting signs what is your differential diagnosis?
(b) What radiographic features can you identify? What is your diagnosis?

194 A grey pony with a heterochromic iris is presented with a swelling of the superior mid-iris region (*Figure 149*).
(a) What is your diagnosis?
(b) What is the differential diagnosis?
(c) What is your treatment?

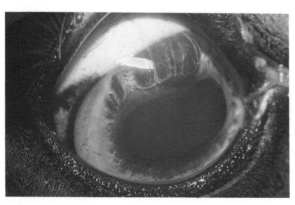

Figure 149

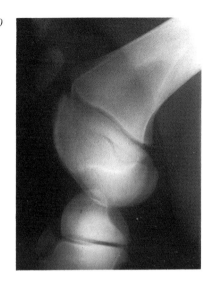

Figure 150

195 A 7-day-old foal presented with left hindlimb lameness associated with distension of the femoropatellar joint capsule. Radiographs of the stifle were obtained.
(a) What views would you obtain?
(b) Describe and explain the radiographic features shown in *Figure 150*.
(c) What is your differential diagnosis?
(d) What additional diagnostic tests would you perform?
(e) When is the patella fully ossified and when does the distal femoral physis close radiographically?

196 A 12-day-old filly has suddenly developed a distended tarsocrural joint capsule (*Figure 151*). She is bright and alert, has a normal body temperature, and is only mildly lame. She is also dripping urine from her umbilicus.
(a) What is your initial diagnostic plan?
(b) What is the most likely diagnosis?
(c) What are the options for therapy?

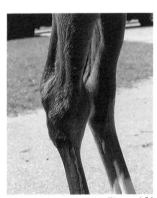

Figure 151

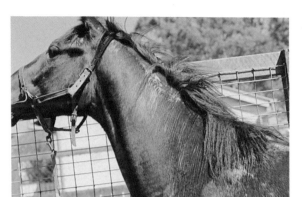

Figure 152

197 A jumping horse returns to training in the spring and is found the following morning to have been rubbing and biting at all parts of his body. Hair has been rubbed or bitten out and the horse is extremely irritable when examined. Rubbed areas occur both under the mane and exposed areas (*Figure 152*).
(a) What are the possible causes?
(b) What treatment would you recommend?

198 A persistent cough with slight unilateral epistaxis had been present in this 12-year-old horse.
(a) Is the lesion illustrated in *Figure 153* responsible for the clinical signs?
(b) What is the diagnosis?
(c) Does the owner have a problem with the horse?

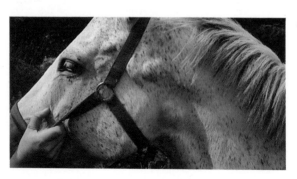

Figure 153

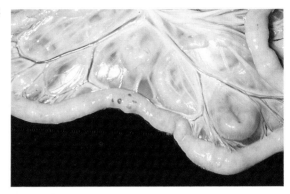

Figure 154

199 The post-mortem appearance of the serosal surface of the small intestine of a yearling Thoroughbred gelding is illustrated in *Figure 154*.
(a) What is the aetiology of the lesion?
(b) What are the possible clinical manifestations of this condition?

Figure 155A

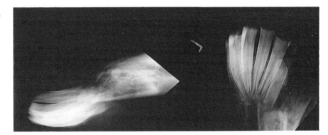

Figure 155B

200 Lateral and intraoral radiographs, illustrated in *Figure 155A*, were obtained from an anaesthetised horse with a suspected fractured mandible (*Figure 155B*).
(a) What are the radiographic findings?
(b) What are the likely clinical findings?
(c) How would you manage this case?

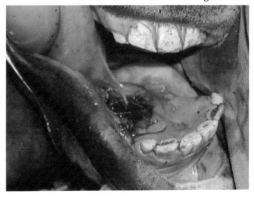

201 What, apart from granulosa cell tumour, are the clinical indications for ovariectomy in mares?

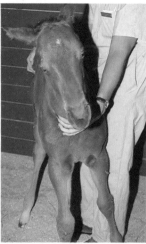

Figure 156

202 The Thoroughbred foal illustrated in *Figure 156* was seen to rear over backwards, striking its poll on a hard surface. It remained recumbent for several minutes and slowly got up showing a right head tilt and right facial paresis and a slightly dysmetric, staggery gait with a tendency to turn to the right.
(a) In addition to these signs, which *one* of the following signs is more likely to be present?
• Central blindness (normal pupils).
• Peripheral blindness (dilated pupils).
• Horner's syndrome (right).
• Masseter atrophy (right).
• Dysphagia.
(b) Why?

203 A 12-hour-old foal is noted by the owner to be rolling (*Figure 157*). Its birth was normal, and it stood and nursed within 2 h of birth. On physical examination, vital signs are within normal limits, but the foal is obviously uncomfortable.
(a) What is the most likely diagnosis?
(b) Do you want to perform any additional diagnostic tests?
(c) What is the treatment of choice?

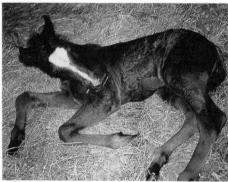

Figure 157

204 Towards the end of the return journey from a competition in Germany a 9-year-old show jumper gelding became colicky, anorexic and dull. Soon after arrival home he was examined. His temperature was 39.5°C, pulse 56/min, (respiration appeared laboured 16 breaths/min). He was depressed, frequently pawed the ground and occasionally looked at his flank. Borborygmi were reduced and per rectum nothing abnormal was palpated. Faeces were dry and scanty.
(a) Describe how you would complete your examination.
(b) From the above information what is a likely diagnosis? What action would you take in terms of treatment and further diagnostic procedures?

205 A 2-month-old colt foal has been deformed since birth (*Figure 158*).
(a) What is the diagnosis?
(b) What is the appropriate treatment?

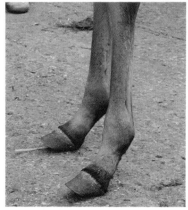

Figure 158

206 *Figure 159* was taken 2 h after the horse had recovered from anaesthesia.
(a) What condition is illustrated?
(b) How should the animal be treated?

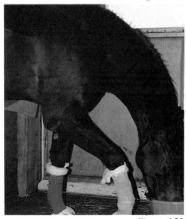

Figure 159

207 An 8-week-old Thoroughbred foal presented with severe left forelimb lameness of acute onset. She tended to stand with the limb partially flexed at the carpus with the elbow 'dropped' and was reluctant to bear weight on the limb when walking, had a markedly shortened cranial phase of the stride and tended to drag the toe as the limb was advanced. There was no detectable crepitus, swelling or focus of pain.

(a) What is your suspected clinical diagnosis?
(b) How would you examine the elbow region radiographically?
(c) Describe the radiographic features shown in *Figure 160*.
(d) Identify A and B in *Figure 160*.
(e) What treatment do you recommend?
(f) When does physeal closure occur radiographically in the ulna and proximal radius? How might this influence case management?

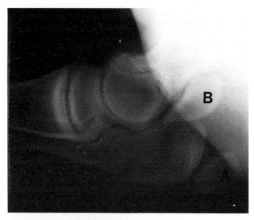

Figure 160

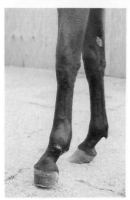

Figure 161

208 The 1-year-old part-bred mare illustrated in *Figure 161* severely injured a fetlock joint at 2 weeks of age.

(a) What clinical signs is she showing?
(b) What is the cause?
(c) What treatment might improve the situation?

209 A 10-year-old three-day-event horse developed right forelimb lameness after the completion of a three-day event. There was distension of both the right and left metacarpophalangeal joint capsules, pain on passive flexion of the joints (right > left) and restricted flexibility. There was diffuse soft-tissue swelling on the proximolateral aspect of the right metacarpophalangeal joint and pain on pressure over the lateral branch of the suspensory ligament.
(a) Describe how to perform an ultrasonographic examination of the suspensory ligament.
(b) Describe the ultrasonographic features shown in *Figures 162A–E*.
(c) What other test(s) or examinations(s) would you perform?

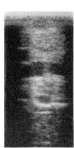

Figure 162A

Figure 162B

Figure 162C

Figure 162D

Figure 162E

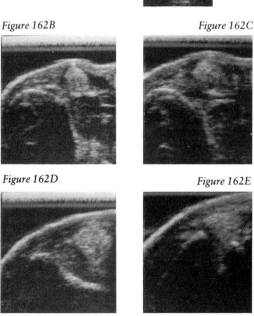

Figure 163

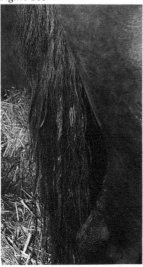

210 The owner of the horse illustrated in *Figure 163* complained that it was lethargic and intermittently lame.
(a) Based on the clinical signs illustrated, has the owner any cause for concern? Can the complaints above be related to these clinical signs?
(b) What is your differential diagnosis?
(c) What further diagnostic tests would be warranted?

211 The owner of a 5-day-old Thoroughbred foal just returns from a vacation and finds him lethargic and tachypnoeic. On physical examination *Figure 164*, you observe the foal to be weak and easily stressed, body temperature is 39.3°C, heart rate 140/min.
(a) What is (are) the first diagnostic test(s) you are going to perform and why?
(b) What is the most likely diagnosis and what are other possibilities?
(c) What treatment is indicated?
(d) What are your recommendations to the owner to try to prevent the same thing from happening again?

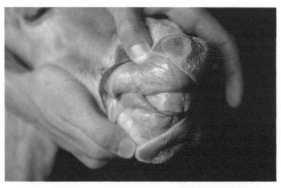

Figure 164

Figure 165

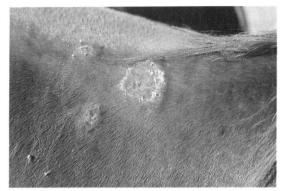

212 A hack is presented with annular scaling lesions on the head, neck and body (*Figure 165*). There is pruritus and previous examinations had failed to demonstrate, either by smear or culture, the presence of pathogenic fungi. Treatment with antiseptics, fungicides and antibiotics by the owner had been unsuccessful.
(a) What is your diagnosis?
(b) What new samples would be necessary to confirm your diagnosis?
(c) What is the most successful treatment?

213 How would you recognise the following during ultrasound scanning of a mare's reproductive tract?
(a) A preovulatory follicle.
(b) Uterine changes which confirm oestrus.
(c) A corpus haemorrhagicum (CH).
(d) A 10-day-old corpus luteum (CL).
(e) A follicle which has luteinised without ovulating.
(f) A mare in prolonged dioestrus.

214 Following the ingestion of some grass cuttings, a 9-year-old pony gelding developed colic characterised by severe unremitting pain. On examination the pony was attempting to roll or 'dog sit' and was sweating. The temperature was 38.5°C, pulse 78/min, respiration 28/min. Mucous membranes were mildly injected. Per rectum the spleen appeared to be displaced caudally. Gas and small amounts of froth were retrieved by stomach tube.
(a) What is wrong with this pony?
(b) How would you manage this case?

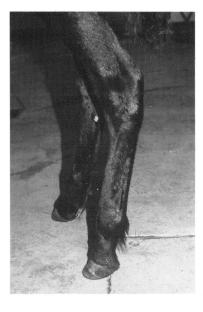

Figure 166

215 The 3-month-old Welsh Cob foal illustrated in *Figure 166* has had an abnormality of its left hindlimb since birth. Note the curby hock appearance.
(a) What may be its cause?
(b) What is the secondary consequence?
(c) What advice should the owner be given?

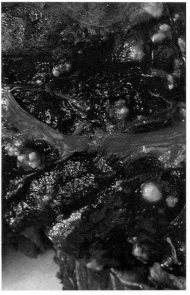

Figure 167

216 The lesions in the liver shown in *Figure 167* were an incidental finding in a horse at post-mortem examination.
(a) What are these lesions?
(b) What is the epidemiology of this condition?
(c) How could the condition have been diagnosed ante-mortem?

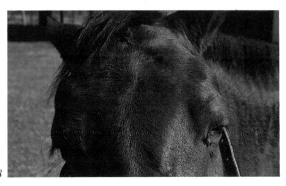

Figure 168

217 The Italian horse illustrated in *Figure 168* was febrile and had extensive limb and ventral abdominal oedema. Three other mares had aborted apparently normal foals over the previous 6–10 days.
(a) What significant signs can be seen?
(b) What diseases should be considered?
(c) If you found diarrhoea, coughing and petechial haemorrhages on the mucous membranes of this horse, which of the possibilities would you consider most likely?

218 The 9-year-old gelding illustrated in *Figure 169* presented with a history of exercise intolerance. Auscultation revealed a resting heart rate of 32 beats/min with second degree atrioventricular (AV) block. A localised grade 2/6 early systolic murmur could be heard over the left heart base, and a grade 2/6 early diastolic murmur could be heard associated with the third heart sound. When exercised the horse showed progressive incoordination of the hindquarters and was extremely distressed.
(a) What is your diagnosis?
(b) What is the likely significance of the cardiac murmurs?
(c) How might you investigate this condition further?
(d) What is the likely prognosis?

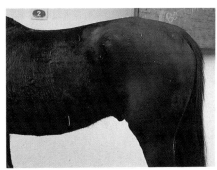

Figure 169. Taken 5 min after a half-mile canter.

219 The investigation of gastrointestinal disturbances in the horse is concerned in the first place with the decision whether the condition requires surgical correction. An immediate prognostic evaluation is also desirable to allow horse owners to balance personal and financial considerations in the decision-making process.

(a) What proportion of colic cases seen in practice require surgical intervention to save the horse's life?

- 5–10%.
- 10–20%.
- 30–50%.

(b) Death as a direct result of colic is usually due to acute cardiovascular failure (shock). What are the overall survival rates of colic surgery in the horse?

- <30%.
- 30–40%.
- 50–60%.
- 70–80%.

(c) What is the average time limit after onset of pain for horses with a strangulation obstruction to stand a reasonable chance of survival after surgery?

- 8 h for small intestine and 4 h for large intestine.
- 4 h for small intestine and 8 h for large intestine.
- 12 h for small intestine and 8 h for large intestine.
- 8 h for both small and large intestine.

(d) Mortality rates are highest for:

- Ileal impaction.
- Large colon torsion of 360°.
- Non-strangulating large colon displacements.
- Small intestinal incarceration into the epiploic foramen.

(e) The most common cause for failure to save the surgical colic horse is:

- The failure to provide adequate fluid therapy.
- The surgeon's skill and experience.
- The failure to decompress the horse's stomach.
- The indiscriminate use of flunixin meglumine (Finadyne).
- The delay in deciding to initiate surgery.

(f) Survival rates are dramatically decreased in colic horses with:

- Heart rate > 100 beats/min.
- PCV > 60%.
- Heart rate 60–80 beats/min and PCV 50–60%.
- Heart rate 80–100 beats/min and PCV < 20%.
- Heart rate > 100 beats/min and PCV > 60%.

Figure 170

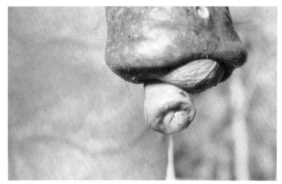

220 A stallion is presented to you with a history of bleeding from the penis after serving mares. You examine the horse's penis and find the urethral process enlarged, containing a cheesy granular-like pus (*Figure 170*). It bleeds very easily when debrided.
(a) What disease process is likely to be present?
(b) What is your differential diagnosis?
(c) How could it be treated?
(d) Is the presence of blood detrimental to the fertility of the stallion's service?

221 An 11-year-old pony mare is suspected of suffering from small intestinal malabsorption because of an 8-week history of rapid weight loss, ventral oedema and low grade abdominal pain. Serum biochemistry has revealed hypoalbuminaemia (albumin 15.3 g/l) in the absence of any other significant abnormalities. An oral glucose tolerance test (performed as described previously) gave the following results:

Time after administration of glucose (min)	Plasma glucose (mmol/l)
0 (pre-administration)	3.8
30	4.8
60	5.1
90	5.5
120	5.9
180	4.0

(a) How do you interpret these results?
(b) What further diagnostic procedures might you use?

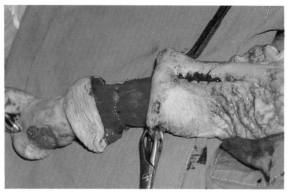

Figure 171

222 A 12-year-old pony gelding presented with a foul-smelling
serosanguinous preputial discharge and oedema.
(a) What lesion is present on the distal body of the penis (*Figure 171*)?
(b) What surgical procedure is being performed (*Figure 171*)?
(c) What are the possible complications of this procedure?
(d) What prognostic indications may be used for the long-term success of this
procedure?
(e) What other surgical procedures may be used to treat this lesion?

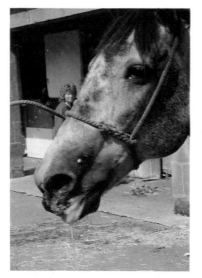

223 The clinical signs illustrated
in *Figure 172* developed gradually
over 3 weeks.
(a) List three significant signs.
(b) What other signs are likely to
have been present associated with
the observed clinical signs?
(c) What diagnostic conclusions
can be drawn from this case?
(d) What further diagnostic tests
would you perform?

Figure 172

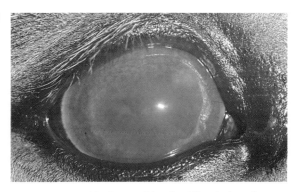

Figure 173

224 A 3-year-old Thoroughbred gelding is thought to have injured an eye (*Figure 173*).
(a) What is your diagnosis?
(b) On what do you base your diagnosis?
(c) What is your treatment?

225 *Figure 174* is the post-mortem appearance of the liver of a 2-year-old donkey.
(a) Identify the organisms in the bile ducts.
(b) What clinical signs might you expect in an animal with this infection?
(c) How could you confirm this condition in the live animal?
(d) What treatment would you recommend for this condition?

Figure 174

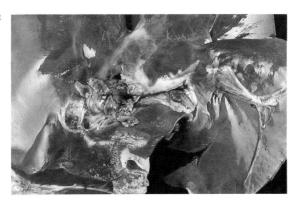

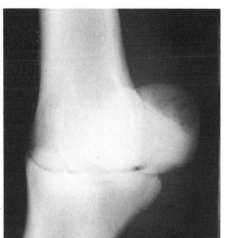

Figure 175

226 The right metacarpophalangeal joint of a 10-year-old event horse (see question **209**) was examined radiographically.
(a) Describe the radiographic features shown in *Figure 175*.
(b) What is the likely significance of your observations?
(c) How would you investigate further?
(d) What is thought to be the cause of the radiographic appearance of the proximal sesamoid bone?

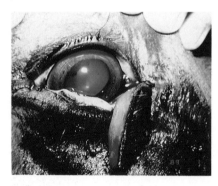

Figure 176

227 A lower eyelid was torn 30 min prior to examination (*Figure 176*).
(a) Should this injury be repaired or the skin flap removed?
(b) What chemical restraint could be used for its repair?
(c) What suture material and suture pattern would you select for:
• Suturing the conjunctiva.
• Skin.

228 The owner of a horse reported a persistent epiphora.
(a) What significant radiographic sign can be seen in *Figure 177*? What is the likely aetiology and outcome?
(b) What further diagnostic procedures should have been performed before radiography to investigate the cause of epiphora?
(c) How are the clinical signs related to the radiographic changes?

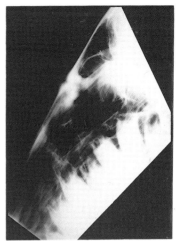

Figure 177

229 A non-pregnant 10-year-old mare which has not exhibited oestrus during June is treated with prostaglandin at the end of the month. What possible reasons can there be for her not subsequently showing signs of oestrus?

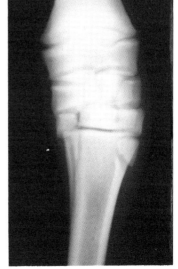

230 A 2-month-old foal has an angular deformity of its left carpus (see radiograph in *Figure 178*).
(a) What is the diagnosis?
(b) What treatment is indicated?
(c) What is the prognosis?

Figure 178

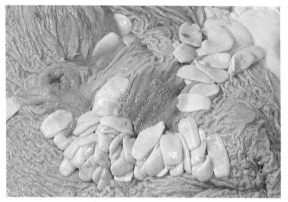

Figure 179

231 *Figure 179* shows the luminal surface of the
caecum of an adult horse.
(a) What intestinal parasites are illustrated?
(b) What is their pathogenic importance?
(c) How would you detect an infection with these
parasites and what treatment would you recommend?

232 A 3-year-old gelding is presented to you with a history of male-like
behaviour, which has included mounting of mares in the paddock in which he
has been kept. What laboratory tests would you use in attempting to confirm
cryptorchid status in this horse?

233 An owner wants information on how much sodium (Na) and calcium
(Ca) they should feed their horse when at rest and in work.
(a) What are the maintenance requirements of Na?
(b) What are the maintenance requirements of Ca?
(c) How much Ca and Na does sweat contain?
(d) How much sweat does an exercising horse produce?
(e) How much Na will an exercising horse require?
(f) How much Ca will an exercising horse require?

234 *Figure 180* illustrates the endoscopic view of the pharynx and larynx of a 5-year-old gelding which had been purchased subject to approval. However, it had shown a bilateral green discharge and abnormal respiratory sounds at exercise. What advice would you give to the potential purchaser?

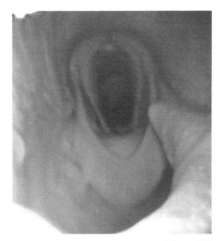

Figure 180

235 (a) What abnormality is shown in *Figure 181* and is it significant?
(b) What other problem might be persistently present?
(c) What acute and chronic conditions might this horse suffer from?
(d) Is there any cure for the behaviour?

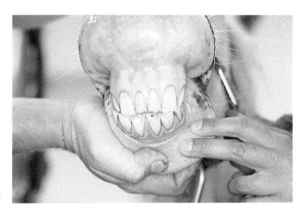

Figure 181

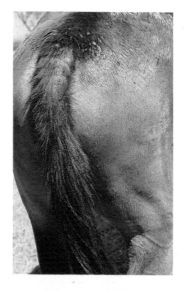

236 A horse is presented to you in mid-summer with a badly rubbed out tail and tail head (*Figure 182*). The horse has been noticed to be constantly rubbing its tail and neck. On examination you find small nodules on the skin over the head, ears, neck, back, croup and tail. Some areas have been rubbed raw, with serum oozing from the rubbed areas.
(a) What is your clinical diagnosis?
(b) What other diseases would you consider, and what are their diagnostic characteristics?

Figure 182

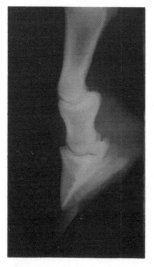

Figure 183A

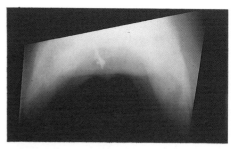

Figure 183B

237 A 12-year-old Thoroughbred mare was severely lame on her left hindlimb (see radiographs in *Figures 183A* and *B*).
(a) For how long is it likely that she has been lame?
(b) What is the cause?
(c) What treatment is indicated?

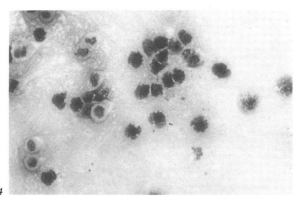

Figure 184

238 A 3-year-old child's pony has been coughing for 3 months, since purchase by the current owners. The pony has been stabled on straw since purchase; before this it was grazing with other horses and a donkey. The pony seems well in all other respects, and has been wormed twice with pyrantel pamoate in the past 8 weeks. The coughing is paroxysmal in nature, and there is no associated nasal discharge or pyrexia. Auscultation of the lungs reveals harsh bronchial sounds only. A transtracheal aspirate has been obtained for cytological examination (*Figure 184*).
(a) What is the likely diagnosis, and how could you confirm this?
(b) How would you treat this pony?

239 The ECG shown in *Figure 185* was obtained from a horse under general anaesthesia.
(a) What type of rhythm is present? (The paper speed is 25 mm/s.)
(b) What is the prognosis for this horse without treatment?
(c) How would you treat this case?

Figure 185

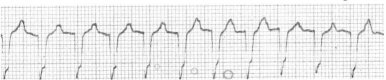

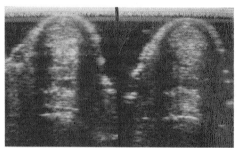

Figure 186

240 An 8-year-old event horse hit a fixed cross-country fence but completed the course, finishing sound. The following day there was diffuse soft-tissue swelling on the dorsal aspect of the right carpus, and mild lameness. Clinical examination also revealed heat in the proximal palmar aspect of the metacarpal region and slight pain on palpation of the margins of the superficial digital flexor tendon.
(a) How do you interpret the ultrasonogram shown in *Figure 186*?
(b) What is your advice?

241 A foal is presented to you on day 2 post-partum. It has difficulty in standing and the dam was observed to have an abnormal discharge at the time of foaling. Clinical examination results in the formation of a preliminary diagnosis of neonatal septicaemia. What clinical pathology aids might be helpful to you, prior to the initiation of treatment?

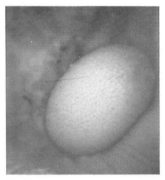

Figure 187

242 *Figure 187* shows a cystoscopic image from a gelding presented with a 12-month history of intermittent haematuria.
(a) What is your diagnosis?
(b) What is the likely composition of the lesion?
(c) How would you surgically manage this case?
(d) What are the potential complications of these procedures?

Figure 188

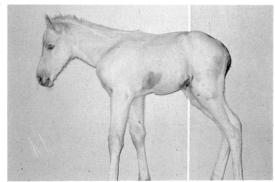

243 An 18-hour-old paint colt, illustrated in *Figure 188*, has not been observed to pass any faeces since birth. He is becoming increasingly colicky, and his abdomen is starting to distend.
(a) What are the most likely differential diagnoses?
(b) What are the most appropriate diagnostic tests?
(c) What is the treatment of choice for the most likely differential?

244 A 4-year-old Highland pony mare had an excessive thirst (~225 l/day) for several months. The pony had normal demeanour, ate well and was in good body condition. The plasma concentrations of urea, creatinine and glucose were within normal ranges in several blood samples from this animal. The results of urinalyses, listed in *Table 3*, were performed on samples obtained before and after deprivation of water for an 18-h period.
(a) What is the probable diagnosis?
(b) Was a water deprivation test appropriate in this case?
(c) What other investigational procedures could be used in this case?

Table 3. Urinalysis results.

	0 h	*+ 18 h* *water deprivation*
Protein (mg/100 ml)	0	0
Glucose (%)	0	0
pH	8.2	8.0
Sp. gr.	1.004	1.008

245 What ultrasonographic uterine features suggest endometritis?

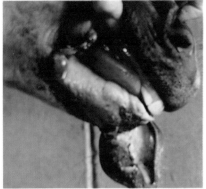

Figure 189

246 A yearling was presented 8 weeks after an injury to its lower lip. The side of the mouth is exposed and a large portion of the lower lip is unattached (*Figure 189*). Discuss the steps taken for its cosmetic and functional repair.

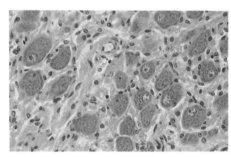

Figure 190A

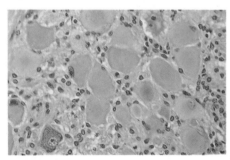

Figure 190B

247 The two histological sections in *Figures 190A* and *B* show nervous tissue taken at post-mortem examination of a normal horse (A) and a case of suspected subacute grass sickness (B) (stain: haematoxylin & eosin; magnification ×235).
(a) Which tissues have been collected in order to confirm the diagnosis?
(b) List the pathological changes in the section from the suspected grass sickness case.
(c) What is your conclusion from these findings?

248   The 12-year-old pony illustrated in *Figure 191* had been suffering from diarrhoea and weight loss for 4 weeks prior to presentation. Small nodules were palpated in the mesentery on rectal examination and the rectal mucosa felt thickened. No other clinical abnormalities were detected. The pony was treated with anthelmintics, antibiotics and antidiarrhoetics but did not improve.

One month later diarrhoea was accompanied by intermittent rectal prolapse. Repeated faecal tests were negative for parasites and significant bacteria. The blood picture was as follows: PCV, 371/l; RBC, 6.7×10^{12}/l; Hb, 11.3 g/dl; WBC 5.2×10^9/l, with 58% neutrophils, 40% lymphocytes and 2% eosinophils. A few atypical lymphocytes with lobed nuclei were seen on smear. TP, 41 g/l; albumin, 19 g/l; globulin, 22 g/l; AST, 136 u/l; GGT, 10 u/l. Histological findings from a rectal biopsy were consistent with chronic colitis. A glucose tolerance test was performed. Basal glucose level was 60 mg/ml; at 1 h it was 60 mg/ml and at 2 and 3 h 70 mg/ml.

(a) From this evidence can you deduce a likely diagnosis?
(b) How would you embark on a diagnostic work up of a chronic weight-loss case?

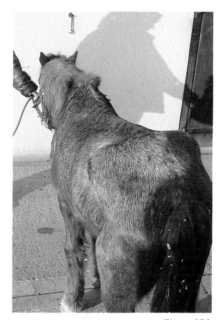

Figure 191

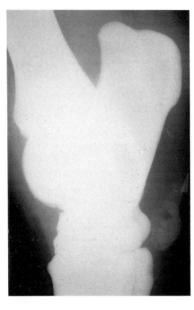

249 A 6-year-old pony mare had intermittent low grade lameness on her right hindlimb.
(a) What abnormality is shown on *Figure 192*?
(b) How might this be investigated further?
(c) What treatment is indicated?

Figure 192

Figure 193

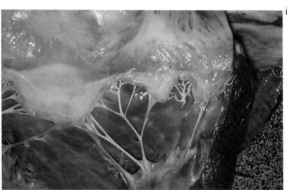

250 *Figure 193* shows the post-mortem appearance of the mitral valve in a 5-year-old Thoroughbred mare.
(a) What does the post-mortem show?
(b) What would be the likely presenting signs?
(c) What is the prognosis for this condition in life?

251 *Figure 194* shows a 15-year-old mare with a parotid swelling which is causing concern to the owner. What is the lesion and how has it arisen?

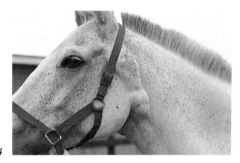

Figure 194

252 A 13-year-old gelding has had a history of chronic weight loss over a 4-month period, to the point that he has become emaciated. His appetite has been capricious, and he has suffered repeated bouts of oesophageal choke. Physical and laboratory examinations have revealed an intermittent, low-grade fever, anaemia, and slight elevation of peritoneal fluid protein content. A mass in the cranial abdomen has been detected by rectal examination.
(a) What condition(s) do you suspect?
(b) How would you confirm your diagnosis?

253 A 2-year-old Thoroughbred colt was presented with a fractured mandible and a swollen left hock (*Figure 195*).
(a) Are the conditions related?
(b) What is the diagnosis?
(c) What advice should be given to the owner?

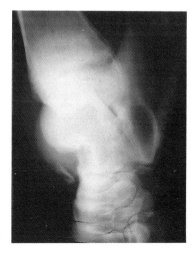

Figure 195

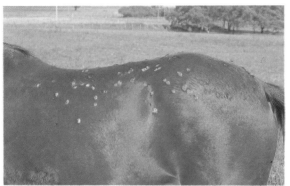

Figure 196

254 A race filly had developed raised hair patches arranged in irregular small groups over her body and neck. The hair plucks with some difficulty, but after a further 7–10 days, most of the hair has fallen out, leaving small annular lesions with a light scurf (*Figure 196*).
(a) What is your diagnosis?
(b) How is the disease spread?
(c) Can the organism survive off the horse?

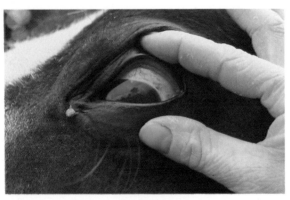

Figure 197

255 (a) Is the clinical sign illustrated in *Figure 197* significant?
(b) What reasons other than infections may be responsible for this?

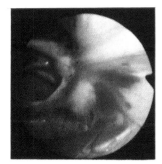

Figure 198A

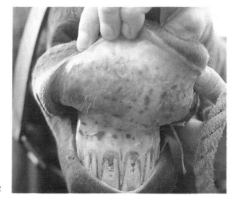

Figure 198B

256 A 5-year-old mare has been undergoing antimicrobial treatment for sinusitis for 10 days when epistaxis develops. A tentative diagnosis of guttural pouch mycosis is made on the basis of endoscopic findings (*Figure 198A*). Is this the typical appearance? What does an oral inspection reveal (*Figure 198B*)? What do you suspect may have happened to the mare?

Figure 199

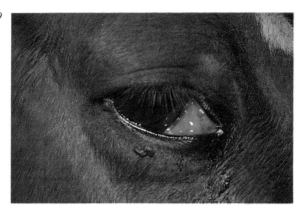

257 An 8-year-old riding horse is presented with swelling of the third eyelid of a few weeks' duration and a persistent ocular discharge, in spite of antimicrobial therapy (*Figure 199*).
(a) What is your clinical diagnosis?
(b) How would you confirm this?
(c) What is your treatment?

258 A frantic owner calls you about a 2-hour-old, 45-kg foal whose mother is dying following the birth process, presumably because of a uterine artery rupture. She anticipates raising the foal as an orphan, and has several questions about the management of this foal. At this time, the foal is standing and appears healthy.
(a) How soon must the foal ingest colostrum?
(b) How can she tell whether the mare's udder contains good quality colostrum?
(c) How much colostrum should the foal ingest and how should she supply it?
(d) How much milk should the foal be ingesting during the first 1–2 weeks of life?
(e) What type of mare milk replacer should she feed the foal?
(f) How can she tell if the foal is taking in sufficient milk?
(g) What veterinary care should the foal receive during the first 24 h of life?

259 How would you advise a stud manager to try to stimulate barren and maiden mares to have ovulatory oestrous periods by late February.

260 The blood biochemical and haematological results in *Table 4* were obtained on analysis of samples from a 9-year-old pony which had a 2-month history of dullness, lethargy and weight loss associated with a poor appetite.
(a) What is the probable diagnosis?
(b) What are the possible causes of this condition?

Table 4

Blood biochemistry	Found	Normal range	Haematology	Found	Normal range
Sodium	130	134–143 mmol/l	Red blood cells	5.8	$6.5–12.5 \times 10^2/l$
Potassium	3.6	3.3–5.3 mmol/l	Packed cell volume	0.30	0.35–0.45 l/l
Chloride	85	89–106 mmol/l	Haemoglobin	11.9	11.0–16.0 g/dl
Calcium	4.3	2.9–3.9 mmol/l	Mean cell volume	36	31.0–41.0 fl
Phosphate	0.4	0.5–1.6 mmol/l	White blood cells	8.9	$4.0–10.0 \times 10^9/l$
Urea	26	3.5–8.0 mmol/l	Neutrophil	6.23	$1.4–5.8 \times 10^9/l$
Creatinine	1150	90–180 µmol/l	Lymphocyte	2.47	$1.4–4.7 \times 10^9/l$
Alkaline phosphatase	196	50–250 mmol/l	Monocyte	0.20	$0–0.2 \times 10^9/l$
Glucose	4.6	3.5–5.9 mmol/l			
Total protein	60	46–70 g/l			
Albumin	24	17–37 g/l			
Globulin	36	21–41 g/l			

261 The febrile horse illustrated in *Figures 200A and B* was presented in Zimbabwe during the rainy season.
(a) What clinical signs are apparent?
(b) What is the likely diagnosis and what is the geographical distribution of this disease?
(c) What epidemiological factors are important?

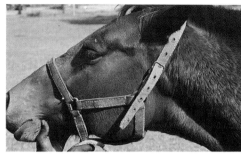

Figure 200A

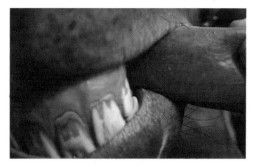

Figure 200B

Figure 201

262 After excessive wet weather, a paddocked horse is noticed to be lame and is found to have a discharging area at the coronary band (*Figure 201*).
(a) What possible conditions could be present?
(b) How can it be treated?

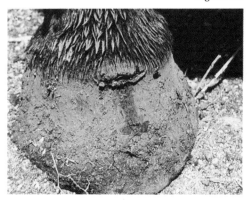

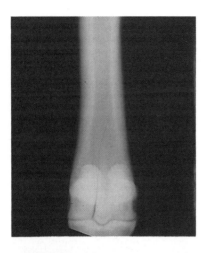

263 A 6-year-old gelding presented with severe lameness, of sudden onset, on his left forelimb (see radiograph in *Figure 202*).
(a) What is the diagnosis?
(b) Is this the most common injury of this type?
(c) What treatment is indicated?

Figure 202

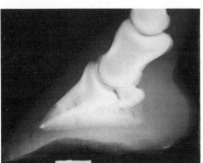

Figure 203A

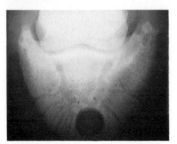

Figure 203B

264 A 5-year-old Warmblood gelding presented with right hindlimb lameness of several weeks' duration. Lameness improved with box rest but recurred with work. The right hindfoot had a slightly longer toe than the left. Lameness was improved by perineural analgesia of the plantar (abaxial sesamoid) nerves.
(a) Describe the radiographic features in *Figures 203A* and *B.*
(b) What is your differential diagnosis?
(c) What treatment would you recommend?
(d) What is your prognosis?

265 A 4-day-old 50-kg foal is presented with a history of watery diarrhoea (*Figure 204*) for the past 18 h. The foal is not interested in nursing, and is becoming increasingly lethargic. WBC count, 3000 cells/μl; fibrinogen, 600 mg/dl; Na^+, 125 mEq/l; K^+, 2.9 mEq/l; Cl^- 93 mEq/l; total CO_2, 15 mEq/l; PCV, 35%; total plasma protein, 7.1 g/dl.

(a) Based on your estimate of the foal's degree of dehydration, how much fluid is required to replace the foal's fluid deficit?

(b) What are the foal's normal (i.e. no increased fluid losses) maintenance fluid requirements?

(c) What type of intravenous fluids would you use to replace the foal's deficits?

(d) What are the most likely causes of diarrhoea in a foal of this age?

(e) What other treatments would you institute at this time?

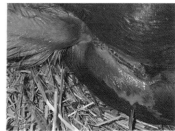

Figure 204

266 The Thoroughbred mare illustrated in *Figure 205* was presented because of an abrupt onset of straining to pass urine and faeces. There was analgesia, areflexia and atonia involving the tail, anus, distal rectum, and perineal skin within the area marked by tape.

(a) Which two diseases should be considered most likely?

(b) Which two of the following are likely to be most contributory to arriving at a clinical diagnosis in each of these two diseases?

- Electromyelography.
- Faecal worm egg count.
- Detailed gait evaluation.
- EHV1 titre.
- Determining if horse has come from North America.
- Rectal examination.
- Cisterna magna CSF analysis.
- Culture for *Listeria*.
- Cranial nerve examination.
- Complete blood count.

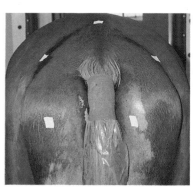

Figure 205

267 A 6-year-old cob gelding is presented with a 2-month history of depression, weight loss and recurrent bouts of colic. The intensity and frequency of the periods of colic have been increasing over the past 2–3 weeks. There appears to be an association between abdominal pain and recent feeding. A full clinical and laboratory work up have failed to identify any significant abnormalities. An oral glucose tolerance test was performed with the following results:

Time after administration of glucose (min)	Plasma glucose (mmol/l)
0 (pre-administration)	4.6
30	4.7
60	4.9
90	7.3
120	9.0
180	9.5
240	9.1

(a) What factors affect the absorptive phase of the test response?
(b) How do you interpret these results?

268 The horse illustrated in *Figure 206* had been dull, off feed and pyrexic at irregular intervals over the past 3 months. Each episode had been treated with a course of antibiotics.
(a) Give two possible causes of these signs.
(b) If several horses had been involved at the same time, which condition would you be most concerned for?
(c) What measures are taken to control this disease?

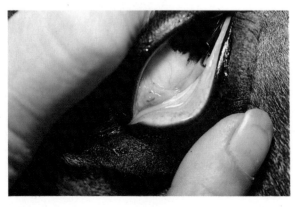

Figure 206

269 *Figure 207* shows the laryngoscopic view from a recently purchased horse. Within 24 h of arriving home the new owner has discovered that exercise provokes harsh inspiratory sounds. What abnormalities can you see and what advice would you give?

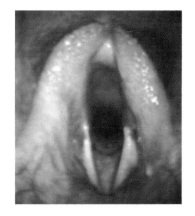

Figure 207

270 A yearling with an injury to the left forelimb (*Figure 208*) was presented following an attempt to jump a gate.
(a) What are the immediate surgical considerations?
(b) What factors will affect healing of this wound?
(c) What surgical techniques might you use to treat this injury?

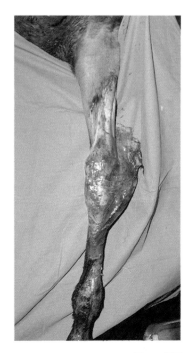

Figure 208

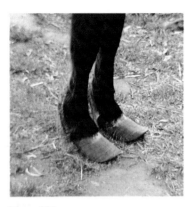

Figure 209

271 A 10-year-old pony is presented with all feet showing overgrowth (*Figure 209*).
(a) What is the condition?
(b) What are the possible causes of the condition?
(c) How can it be treated?

272 An 18-year-old hunter gelding has been subjected to exploratory laparotomy and surgical removal of 4.9 m of jejunum after a small intestinal hernia into the epiploic foramen. The animal made a good anaesthetic recovery and appeared bright during the first 12 h after surgery. It was allowed to satisfy its thirst gradually. Immediately after recovery it had a pulse rate of 60/min and a PCV of 43%. Twelve hours later signs of discomfort were first noticed and a pulse rate of 80/min and a PCV of 52% were registered. Gut sounds were absent and 7 l of gastric reflux were retrieved on nasogastric intubation. Intravenous fluid therapy was started and nasogastric intubation performed every 4 h. This resulted each time in the retrieval of between 2 and 8 l of dark-brown, foul-smelling fluid. After intubation the animal was more comfortable and its pulse rate dropped slightly. The PCV (50%) was kept stable with intravenous fluids. Twenty-four hours later distended loops of small intestine were first detected by palpation per rectum. The distension increased gradually over the next 24 h. Heart rate and PCV were now consistently high (80 beats/min and 55%) and the animal dull and depressed.
(a) What is your diagnosis?
(b) What factors may lead to this condition?
(c) How will you manage the condition medically?
(d) Which surgical alternative is available if medical treatment fails? At what point is surgery indicated?

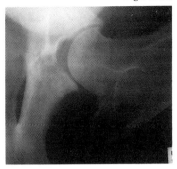

Figure 210

273 A 5-year-old Thoroughbred gelding, with marked muscle atrophy in the right gluteal region, had been lame on its right hindlimb for 9 months prior to this radiographic investigation (*Figure 210*).
(a) What is the diagnosis?
(b) What advice should be given to the owner?

274 A 4-year-old horse in training has had laryngeal surgery during which it was maintained on halothane anaesthesia. It appeared to make a good initial recovery but it has remained inappetent and depressed and there is no evidence of a febrile response. An initial blood biochemistry check taken 14 days postoperatively has demonstrated elevated AST, GGT and GLDH levels. What additional samples would be of value in diagnosis and prognosis?

275 The lesions illustrated in *Figure 211* were of concern to a prospective purchaser of this 8-year-old horse.
(a) Are the lesions likely to cause any clinical problem?
(b) What reassurance can be given to the purchaser?
(c) If the horse had been presented with dysphagia could it be attributed to the clinical signs illustrated?

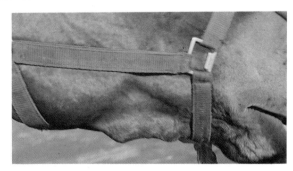

Figure 211

276 What ultrasonographic features would you expect in the uterus of a pregnant mare on the following days after ovulation?
(a) 14 days?
(b) 18 days?
(c) 21 days?
(d) 26 days?
(e) 30 days?
(f) 37 days?
(g) 42 days?
(h) 60 days?
(i) 100 days?

277 The calculus shown in *Figure 212* was removed from the bladder of a 10-year-old mare which was presented for investigation of intermittent haematuria.
(a) What other clinical signs might you have expected to see in this case?
(b) How would you confirm the diagnosis?
(c) How would you manage such a case?

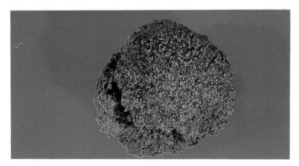

Figure 212

278 A horse with suspected liver disease gave the following result for a Bromosulphthalein (BSP) dye clearance test:

Case	Normal
3.9 (min ($t_{1/2}$))	2.0–3.7

(a) Describe the rationale behind the use of the BSP dye clearance test as an assessment of equine hepatic function.
(b) How would you interpret this result?
(c) Which factors, other than liver disease, can affect the results of this test?

279 A 1-day-old foal is presented with nasal reflux of milk whenever it sucks from the mare. It is also severely dyspnoeic. A tentative diagnosis of cleft palate has been made.
(a) How would you investigate further?
(b) Are there any other possibilities?

280 A horse has recently attended a gymkhana and was obliged to be ridden with a borrowed saddle and fittings; approximately 10 days later a skin eruption occurred around the left girth area showing scurfiness and loss of hair (*Figure 213*).
(a) What is girth itch?
(b) What samples would you take to reach a diagnosis?
(c) What culture method could be used for isolation?
(d) How would you treat the condition?

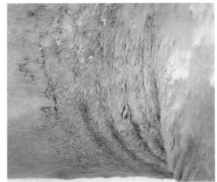

Figure 213

281 A 10-year-old part-bred Arab gelding has chronic swelling in the left stifle region but no obvious lameness (see radiograph shown in *Figure 214*).
(a) What is your differential diagnosis?
(b) What treatment might you suggest?

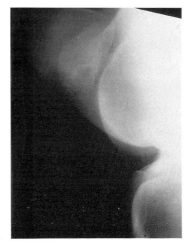

Figure 214

282 Acute salmonellosis is suspected in a yearling cob filly which had undergone general anaesthesia and exploratory laparotomy for the treatment of colic due to small intestinal intussusception 2 days earlier. The filly developed profuse diarrhoea with fever and severe depression.
(a) What basic pathophysiological abnormalities are expected in acute salmonellosis?
(b) How would you monitor the course of the disease and response to treatment?

283 The ECG shown in *Figure 215* was taken from a 12-year-old Thoroughbred mare immediately after exercise.
(a) What abnormalities can be detected?
(b) What is the likely origin of these abnormalities?
(c) What is the likely prognosis in this case?

Figure 215. Lead Z, paper speed 25 mm/sec.

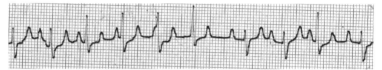

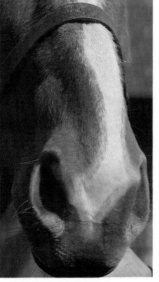

284 A swelling has developed in the subcutaneous tissues 5–7 cm caudal to the upper margin of the nostril (*Figure 216*). The lesion is quite firm on palpation and does not appear to cause discomfort. What is the likely nature of the swelling and what treatment would you suggest?

Figure 216

285 An old wire injury to the bulb of the heel has healed well and the horse has been put back into work, but shows lameness when worked. Examination shows a deep crack still present in the wall (*Figure 217*).
(a) Why is the horse lame?
(b) Can it be cured?
(c) Will the treatment be permanent?
(d) Are there any other treatment options?

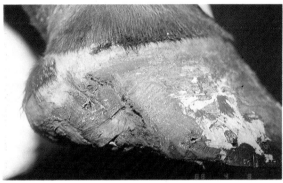

Figure 217

286 A 12-year-old Standardbred gelding was slightly lame on the left forelimb at the trot. The lameness was abolished by palmar digital nerve blocks, following which the animal was slightly lame on the right forelimb.
(a) On the basis of this clinical information, what is the likely diagnosis?
(b) Is the radiograph (*Figure 218*) diagnostic?
(c) What is the diagnosis?

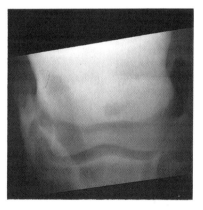

Figure 218

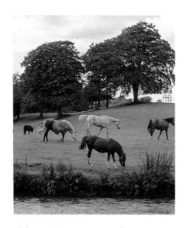

Figure 219

287 A group of eight horses and ponies which are used for pleasure riding are grazed year-round on 4.86 hectares (12 acres) of permanent pasture (*Figure 219*). During the last 4 years these animals have received prophylactic doses of fenbendazole at a rate of 7.5 mg/kg at 2-monthly intervals. The animals are in good physical condition and none have shown clinical signs of disease attributable to parasitic infections.
(a) What are the possible problems which might arise as a consequence of the worming programme?
(b) How might you investigate the efficacy of the worming programme?

288 For what reasons might a multiple (usually twin) pregnancy be missed during ultrasound scanning?

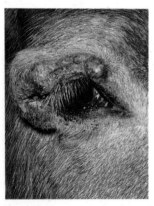

Figure 220

289 A grey pony presents with a swelling involving both upper and lower eyelids (*Figure 220*).
(a) What is the differential diagnosis?
(b) What is the most likely diagnosis and why?
(c) How would you confirm the diagnosis?

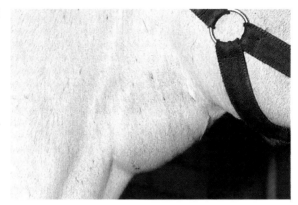

Figure 221

290 A 19-year-old hunter was in good body condition and worked regularly. A firm, smooth, discrete, mobile, subcutaneous swelling in the ventral aspect of the upper neck had been present for several years and the mass had slowly increased in size (*Figure 221*).
(a) What is the probable diagnosis?
(b) How would you confirm this diagnosis?
(c) What treatment would you institute in this case?

291 A 3-year-old Thoroughbred mare had recently gone suddenly lame on her left forelimb.
(a) What is the diagnosis (see radiograph shown in *Figure 222*)?
(b) What treatment is indicated?

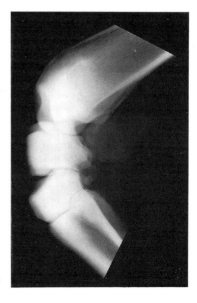

Figure 222

292 A 5-year-old racehorse is presented with a group of variable 5–20 mm subcutaneous nodules over the thorax (*Figure 223*). They have been present for several weeks, appear to be growing in number rather than size, are firm, well demarcated, non-pruritic, non-painful and non-alopecic.
(a) What are the various terms used to describe this disease?
(b) Generally speaking, they are fibrous nodules, but several are very hard; why?
(c) What treatment may be successful?

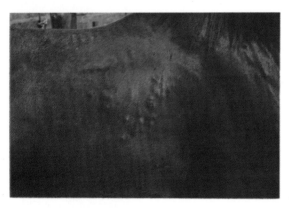

Figure 223

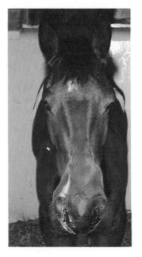

293 The horse illustrated in *Figure 224* presented with these acute signs. Two small puncture wounds on the muzzle were found on close examination.
(a) What significant features can be identified?
(b) List four possible conditions which might present with similar signs.
(c) Is this horse likely to die?

Figure 224

294 A 6-year-old pleasure horse gelding presented with poor hindlimb action of at least several months' duration. The horse had a rather large hock angle (i.e. straight hocks) and demonstrated poor hindlimb impulsion. When the horse was ridden mild left hindlimb lameness predominated. Following subtarsal analgesia of the left hindlimb the horse showed mild right hindlimb lameness.

(a) What further examinations would you perform?
(b) How do you interpret the ultrasonograms (*Figure 225A, B*)?
(c) Describe the radiographic features shown in *Figure 225C and D*.
(d) What is your diagnosis and prognosis?

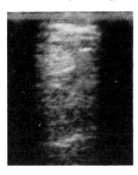

Figure 225A

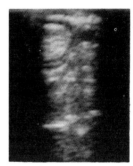

Figure 225B

Figure 225C

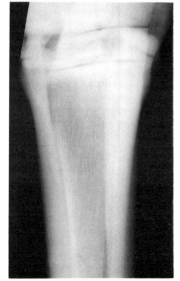

Figure 225D

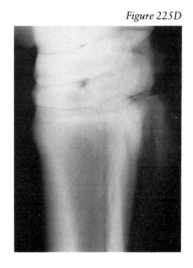

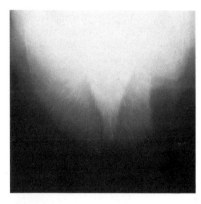

295 A 17-year-old hunter mare had been slightly lame for 4½ months before the radiograph shown in *Figure 226* was obtained. The problem was diagnosed as pus in the foot, but this had not responded to drainage.
(a) What radiographic signs are present?
(b) What is the differential diagnosis?
(c) What advice should be given to the owner?

Figure 226

296 How do you help an owner who wishes to know:
(a) What books are available on equine nutrition?
(b) Where practical information and advice can be obtained on pasture management?
(c) Where practical information and advice can be obtained on feeding regimens?
(d) What cautionary advice is there regarding nutritional dietary requirements?

297 During an examination for purchase the teeth of the horse illustrated in *Figure 227* were inspected to assess its age and its oral conformation. What is the significance of the pattern of wear on the central incisors?

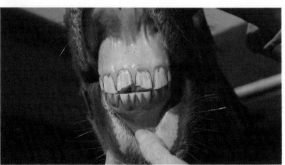

Figure 227

298 (a) What is the diagnosis of the clinical feature shown in *Figure 228*?
(b) Should this horse be ridden?

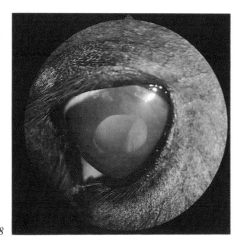

Figure 228

299 A Thoroughbred foal, born 24 h prior to initial presentation, has been noted to be weak and to have a rapid respiratory rate. Clinical examination demonstrates icteric mucous membranes. Your provisional diagnosis of neonatal isoerythrolysis appears to be confirmed by laboratory results indicating severe anaemia and a grossly elevated bilirubin level. Outline your approach to initial treatment.

300 A horse is presented for an extensive skin graft (*Figure 229*). Name three types of grafts which could be used and list their advantages and disadvantages.

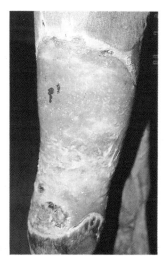

Figure 229

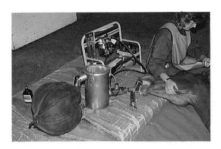

Figure 230A

301 Two types of anaesthetic breathing circuits used in equine anaesthesia are illustrated in *Figures 230A* and *B*.
(a) What types of breathing systems are they examples of?
(b) List their advantages and disadvantages.

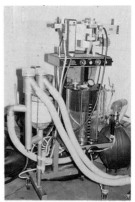

Figure 230B

302 You are asked to examine a mare on a hunter stud in mid-April because she has been at stud for 3 weeks and hasn't been seen in oestrus. What are the possible reasons for this?

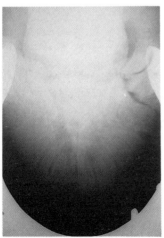

303 An 8-year-old part-bred gelding had been lame for nearly 1 year on his left forelimb. Intra-articular analgesia of the metacarpophalangeal (fetlock) joint abolished the lameness.
(a) What is the diagnosis (see radiograph shown in *Figure 231*)?
(b) What further radiographic investigations are indicated?

Figure 231

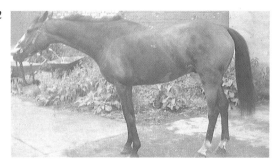

Figure 232

304 The owner of the 8-year-old riding horse illustrated in *Figure 232* reported that the horse had become very colicky on returning from hard exercise. This was manifest by continuous pawing and profuse sweating. When examined 1.5 h after onset, pulse was 60/min and respiration 32/min. Temperature was 38.6°C. Bowel sounds were depressed and mucous membranes mildly injected. Moving his hindquarters seemed painful.
(a) Describe your clinical examination and its relevance to the differential diagnoses you would be considering.
(b) What do you think is the most likely diagnosis?
(c) How would you treat this horse?

305 A 3-month-old foal was presented with a slight purulent nasal discharge and an intermittent pyrexia of 2 weeks' duration.
(a) What significant features can you identify in the radiograph shown in *Figure 233*?
(b) Is this a congenital disease/abnormality?
(c) What is the diagnosis and what other clinical signs may be seen?
(d) What treatment is indicated?

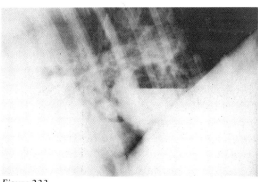

Figure 233

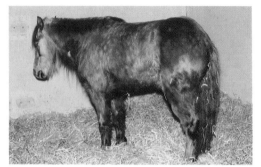

Figure 234

306 A 12-year-old pony mare with ragwort (*Senecio jacobaea*) poisoning showed progressive depression and restlessness over 1 week. Most of her time was spent standing in the position shown in *Figure 234*.
(a) What behaviour is the pony showing and what is this syndrome called?
(b) What are the pathogenic mechanisms resulting in these clinical signs?
(c) How can this aspect of hepatic disease be treated?

307 *Figure 235* is a lateral thoracic radiograph of a 7-year-old gelding which had been observed to have intermittent haematuria for 5 months. During the latter 2 months of illness the animal had been increasingly anorexic with an associated, marked weight loss. Hyperpnoea was evident and on auscultation there was a bilateral absence of lung sounds in the ventral thorax.
(a) What radiological abnormalities are illustrated?
(b) What further diagnostic procedures would you consider appropriate in the investigation of this case?

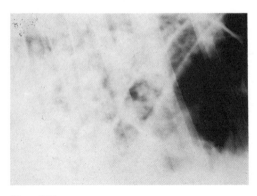

Figure 235

Figure 236

308 A yearling being prepared for a sale is found with a soft cold swelling around the nose and eyes (*Figure 236*). The swelling is not painful and the colt appears bright and alert with normal temperature, pulse and respiration, and is still wanting to eat.
(a) What conditions could be present?
(b) What treatment is likely to be effective?
(c) Would you expect the condition to be recurrent?

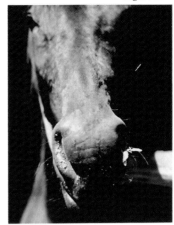

309 The horse illustrated in *Figure 237* had undergone abdominal surgery for the correction of a large bowel displacement. Three days after the surgery he was pyrexic.
(a) What is the likely diagnosis?
(b) What precautions should be taken?
(c) What is the prognosis?

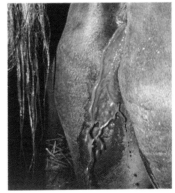

Figure 237

310 A 7-year-old hunter mare has had a 2-year history of mild coughing (mainly in the mornings and at exercise) and intermittent, bilateral mucoid nasal discharge. The coughing is generally only a problem during the winter-time, when the horse is stabled. You are asked to examine her one evening when she was found in her stable, 2 h after being brought in from the field, in severe respiratory distress. Her respiratory rate is 30/min. She is coughing and showing marked inspiratory and expiratory dyspnoea, with flaring of the nostrils and protrusion of the anus with each expiration. The rectal temperature is 39.0°C. Auscultation of the chest reveals widespread crackling and whistling lung sounds.
(a) What is your diagnosis?
(b) How would you treat the mare?

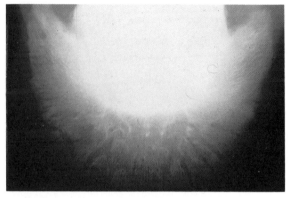

Figure 238

311 An 11-year-old Thoroughbred gelding, in poor condition, had a voracious appetite, and had subsequently become lame.
(a) What lesions are present in the radiograph shown in *Figure 238*?
(b) What is a possible cause?
(c) What further radiographic investigation is indicated?

312 A 4-day-old colt is presented with abdominal distension and lethargy. The body temperature is 39.5°C, the heart rate is 140 beats/min, the respiratory rate 36 breaths/min. Fluid is detected by abdominal wall ballottement. The WBC count is 3600 cells/µl, 60% segmented neutrophils, 10% bands, 30% lymphocytes, fibrinogen 600 mg/dl. Small amounts of foetid diarrhoea are noted. The colt is experiencing increasing pain, and is refractory to analgesic therapy.
(a) What further diagnostic tests are indicated at this time?
(b) What are the most likely differential diagnoses?
(c) What therapy is indicated?

313 *Figure 239* illustrates the traditional technique for dental extraction in the horse, i.e. trephination over the tooth root followed by repulsion. What are the potential complications of this technique?

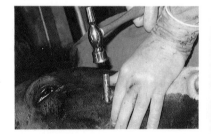

Figure 239

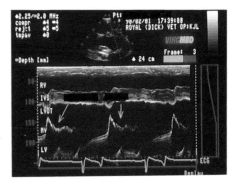

Figure 240A. Right ventricle (RV); interventricular septum (IVS); left ventricular outflow tract (LVOT); mitral valve (MV); left ventricle (LV).

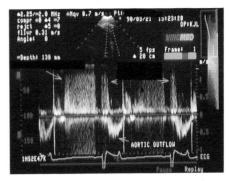

Figure 240B

314 A 15-year-old hunter presented with a grade 3/6 decrescendo diastolic murmur which was audible on both sides of the thorax. It could be heard most clearly over the area of maximum intensity of the second heart sound. The murmur had a buzzing musical component and increased in intensity after the fourth heart sound. The spectral Doppler and M-mode studies from this case are shown in *Figures 240A* and *B*.

(a) What is the cause of this murmur?

(b) What do the M-mode and the spectral Doppler studies show?

(c) What changes would you expect to feel in the facial pulse in more severe cases?

(d) The work history of this horse is good and the owner is keen to continue to ride it. What would you advise?

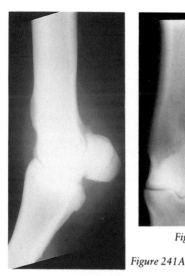

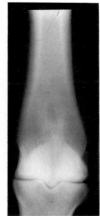

Figure 241B

Figure 241A

315 A 7-year-old gelding had had an injury to the dorsal aspect of its left hindlimb, just above the fetlock joint, 2 months before the radiographs shown in *Figures 241A* and *B* were obtained. The wound had failed to heal completely.
(a) What is the diagnosis?
(b) What treatment is indicated?

316 A horse has developed a skin condition over a period, initially involving the face and neck and now spreading to the trunk (*Figure 242*). The skin displayed seborrhoea and folding, with crusts and scales. There were also lesions around the coronet.
(a) Which group of skin diseases might you investigate?
(b) What specimens are necessary to assist making a diagnosis?
(c) What type of cells would you expect to find in a direct smear from an intact vesicle or pustule on recent erosion?

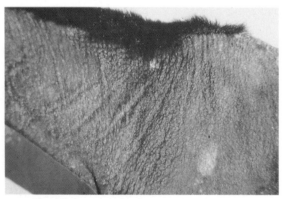

Figure 242 (courtesy of Mr M. Hillyer, University of Bristol)

317 At what stage of pregnancy is the blood test eCG (= PMSG) applicable. What is the cause of false positives?

318 The worm eggs shown in *Figure 243* were identified by flotation of faecal samples from a group of newly weaned pony foals.
(a) Identify the parasitic eggs.
(b) Is infection with these parasites likely to be of clinical significance in these animals?

Figure 243

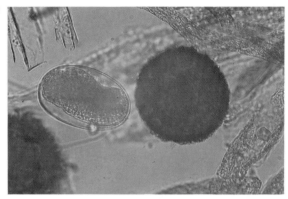

319 A polo pony is presented with a persistent ocular discharge a few weeks after trauma to the eye (*Figure 244*).
(a) What is your diagnosis?
(b) Name two other causes of this condition.
(c) How would you treat this condition?

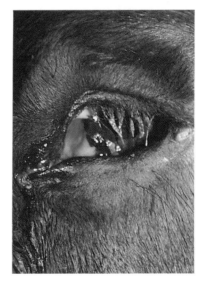

Figure 244

320 The same colt as in
question **44**. Lameness was
improved but not alleviated by
intra-articular analgesia of the
shoulder joint. Radiographic
examination was performed
(*Figure 245*).
(a) Describe the radiographic
features.
(b) What is the differential
diagnosis?
(c) What other diagnostic tests
would you perform?
(d) What treatment would you
recommend?

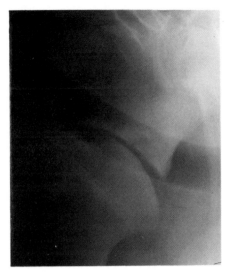

Figure 245

321 A 3-year-old colt in training was presented for investigation of a mild
intermittent cough of 6 days' duration. The horse was not febrile.
(a) Is the clinical sign shown in *Figure 246* significant?
(b) What diagnostic measures would be helpful?
(c) The trainer asks that an antibiotic be administered – would you agree that
such a course is warranted?

Figure 246

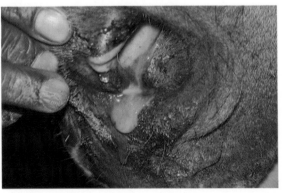

322 A chronic fibrous swelling has occurred over 18 months of poor healing, self-mutilation and incorrect treatment (*Figure 247*).
(a) How could this swelling be treated to achieve a better result?
(b) After your treatment, the horse tries to bite the area; how can this be prevented?

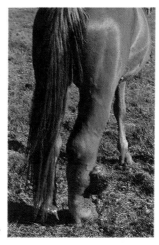

Figure 247

323 A 10-year-old small pony mare was suffering from chronic laminitis, and had a stilted gait on all four feet (see radiographs in *Figure 248*).
(a) What is the diagnosis?
(b) How long is the problem likely to have been present?
(c) What breed is the pony likely to be?

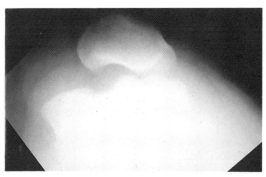

Figure 248

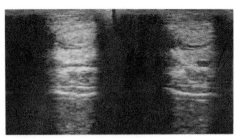
Figure 249

324 A 6-year-old event horse presented with acute onset, moderate left forelimb lameness. No significant palpable abnormalities were identified. Lameness was not improved by perineural analgesia of the palmar digital, palmar (abaxial sesamoid) or palmar (mid-cannon) and palmar metacarpal nerves, but was substantially improved by subcarpal analgesia.
(a) What additional examinations would you perform?
(b) Describe the ultrasonographic features shown in *Figure 249*.
(c) What is your diagnosis? What might you do to substantiate it?
(d) What is your treatment and prognosis?

325 The only neurological signs the foal illustrated in *Figure 250* is demonstrating are slight ptosis and miosis and sweating on the face and neck down to the level of C2 as shown. Which of the following combination of interpretations of the lesion and the causative disease is most likely correct?
- Preganglionic cervical sympathetic lesion; neck abscess.
- Oculomotor paralysis; equine protozoal myeloencephalitis.
- Facial paralysis; head trauma.
- Horner's syndrome; postganglionic sympathetic neuropathy.
- Cranial nerve V and VII involvement; guttural pouch empyema.

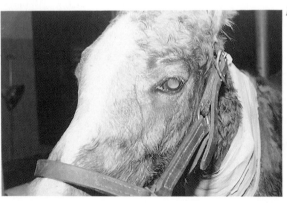
Figure 250

326 A 4-year-old Arab gelding had been slightly lame on its left forelimb for 2 months.
(a) Is the radiograph shown in *Figure 251* diagnostic?
(b) What further investigations might be useful?
(c) What advice should be given to the owner?

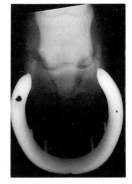

Figure 251

327 A 7-year-old show jumper mare presented with moderate left hindlimb lameness of several weeks' duration. There was moderate enlargement of the digital flexor tendon sheaths in the fetlock regions of both hindlimbs (windgalls), more marked in the left than the right. In both limbs there was slight indentation at the level of the plantar annular ligaments. Flexion of the hock did not alter the gait but lameness was accentuated by flexion of the distal limb joints. Lameness persisted after perineural analgesia of the plantar (abaxial sesamoid) nerves but was improved by perineural analgesia of the plantar (mid-cannon) and plantar metatarsal nerves.
(a) What additional diagnostic tests would you perform?
(b) How do you interpret the ultrasonograph shown in *Figure 252*?
(c) What is your diagnosis, treatment and prognosis?

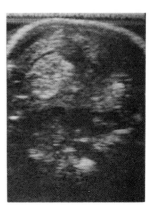

Figure 252

328 A colt foal weighing 59.5 kg at birth is presented to you on the third day post-partum. It appears to strain on attempting to urinate and voids small volumes of urine, frequently. What samples could be submitted to a clinical pathology laboratory to confirm a provisional diagnosis of uroperitoneum?

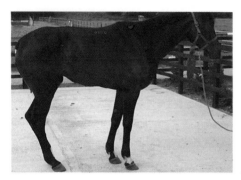

329 The 4-year-old horse illustrated in *Figure 253* had chronic grass sickness which was confirmed at post-mortem. What are the most reliable clinical signs?

Figure 253

330 A foal was apparently normal until 2 h old, when the owners noted him to be slightly lethargic and the mare's udder somewhat distended. At 48 h of age capillary refill time is 2.5 s, pulse quality is fair, body temperature 38.8°C, WBC count 4000 cells/μl. The serum IgG concentration is 200–400 mg/dl, by a field test.
(a) What is the most likely diagnosis (refer to *Figure 254*)?
(b) What additional diagnostic tests would you perform to confirm this diagnosis?
(c) What therapy are you going to institute?

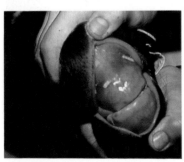

Figure 254

331 A 13-year-old mare was 10 months pregnant. She had been showing moderate occasionally severe colic signs for 2 h. Faecal production was reduced and borborygmi depressed but present. Pulse was 48/min, respiration 20/min. What are the main differential diagnoses and what are their distinguishing features? How would you treat them?

332 A mare spontaneously delivers a 25-kg Arabian filly at 305 days' gestation, 2 weeks after mammary development and spontaneous lactation began. The foal is weak after birth, and body temperature at 2 h old is 37.7°C. The heart rate is 100 beats/min, pulses are strong, and respiratory rate is 50 breaths/min, with a slightly increased abdominal effort. A grade III/VI holosystolic murmur is auscultated at the third intercostal space on the left side. The WBC count is 9000 cells/μl, fibrinogen is 800 mg/dl, and the pH is 7.386, P_{CO_2} 49 mmHg, P_{O_2} 45 mmHg, HCO_3^- 27 mEq/l, at 2 h of age.
(a) What respiratory supportive care is indicated at this time?
(b) What is the most likely diagnosis (refer to *Figures 255A* and *B*)?
(c) What other therapeutic measures are indicated at this time?
(d) What advice can you give the owner regarding the short- and long-term prognosis for this animal (assuming intensive critical care is available and is economically feasible)?

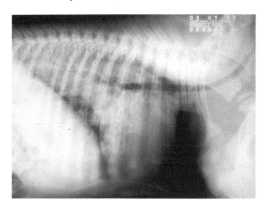

Figure 255A

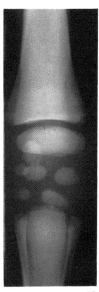

Figure 255B

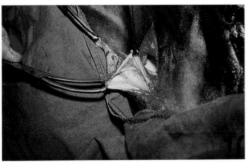

333 A surgical incision has been made in the scrotal region of a cryptorchid horse and the margins of the superficial inguinal ring have been identified. A structure consisting of a tube of white fibrous tissue partially covered by striated muscle has been identified within the inguinal canal. This structure has been incised and the contents exposed. Its tip is held by one

Figure 256

pair of forceps and the cut margins by other forceps, thus exposing the contents, a solid band of fibrous tissue.

(a) What is the tube-like structure and its accompanying muscle?
(b) Why is it important to identify this structure during inguinal exploration of the inguinal region of a cryptorchid horse?
(c) What possible structures could be found inside the tube-like structure?
(d) Which of these possibilities is demonstrated in the picture?

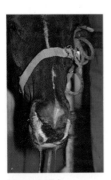

Figure 257A

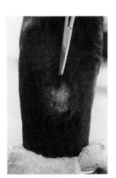

Figure 257B

334 The horse illustrated in *Figure 257A* was presented for examination in Central Africa. The horse persistently bit at its left knee where a shallow wound was present (*Figure 257B*). A mild hindlimb ataxia progressed over a period of 4 days to recumbency and terminated after 5 days in convulsions and coma.

(a) What disease should be considered first?
(b) How may this be confirmed?
(c) What measures should be taken by persons in contact with the animal.

335 The foal described in question **332** is now 4 days old, having responded well to your treatment. You noted that urine output suddenly decreased 12 h earlier, and now the foal appears slightly more lethargic. Serum electrolytes are as follows: Na^+ 120 mEq/l, K^+ 5.2 mEq/l, Cl^- 90 mEq/l, serum creatinine 2.0 mg/dl. Based on the history and your ultrasound examination of the abdominal cavity (*Figure 258*):
(a) What is the most likely diagnosis?
(b) What test would you run to confirm your diagnosis?
(c) What type of fluid replacement therapy is indicated at this time?

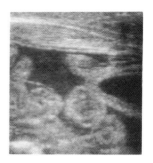

Figure 258

336 *Figure 259* illustrates a horse being prepared for general anaesthesia to allow surgical correction of a suspected high small intestinal obstruction.
(a) What procedure is illustrated?
(b) Why is this important prior to the proposed anaesthetic and surgery?

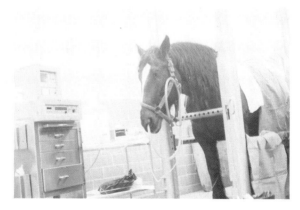

Figure 259

ANSWER ILLUSTRATIONS

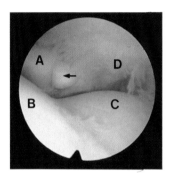

Figure 260. Dorsoproximal articular surface, proximal phalanx (A); sagittal ridge, third metacarpal bone (B); medial condyle, third metacarpal bone (C); synovial membrane (D); osteochondral fragment (arrow).

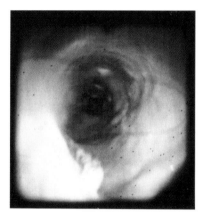

Figure 261

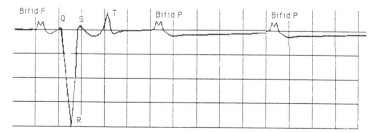

Figure 262

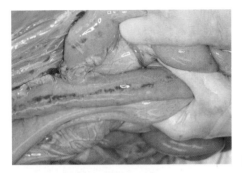

Figure 263

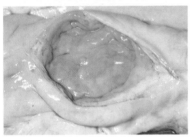

Figure 264A

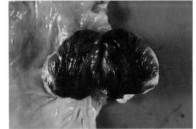

Figure 264B

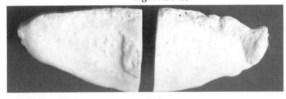

Figure 265

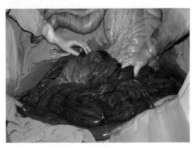

Figure 266A. Discoloured bowel with
mesenteric haemorrhage and
thrombosis.

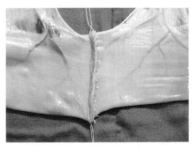

Figure 266B. Everting mattress suture.

160

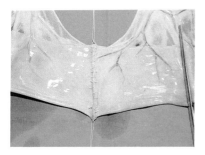

Figure 266C. Opposing simple interrupted suture.

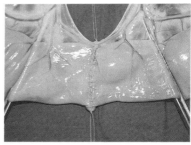

Figure 266D. Inverted interrupted Lembert suture.

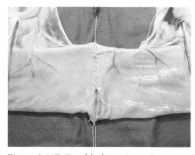

Figure 266E. Double-layer inverting closure (simple interrupted plus continuous Lembert).

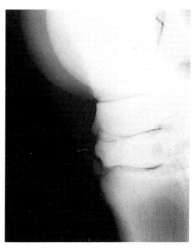

Figure 267

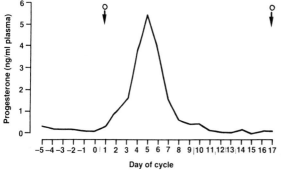

Figure 268

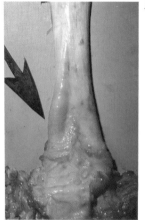

Figure 269

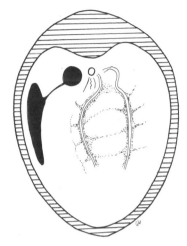

Figure 271A. Rectal findings.

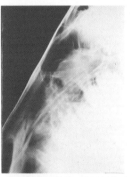

Figure 270A

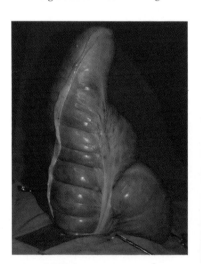

Figure 271B. Laparotomy reveals a
grossly enlarged tympanic caecum.

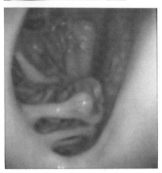

Figure 270B

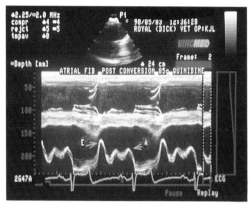

Figure 272

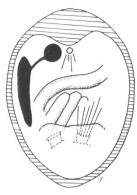

Figure 273. Rectal findings.

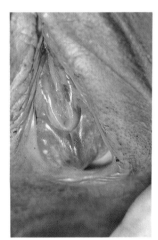

Figure 274A

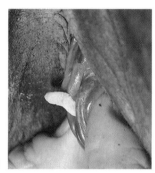

Figure 274B

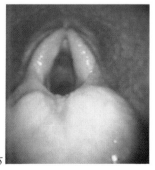

Figure 275

163

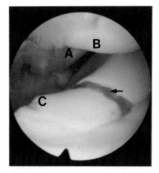

Figure 276. Medial condyle, third metacarpal bone (A); sagittal ridge, third metacarpal bone (B); apex medial sesamoid bone (C); fracture plane (arrow).

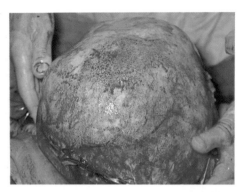

Figure 277A

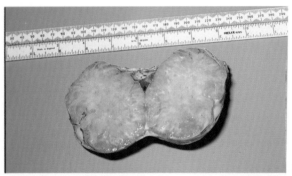

Figure 277B

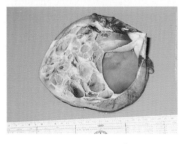

Figure 277C

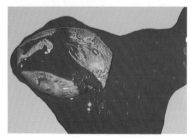

Figure 277D

164

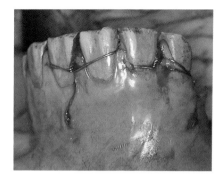

Figure 278

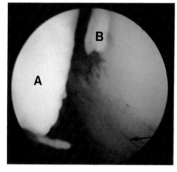

Figure 279. Displaced fracture (A); comminution (B); wear lines (arrow).

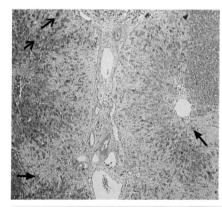

Figure 280. Photomicrograph of a section of liver from a case of ragwort poisoning showing loss of hepatocytes and replacement with fibrous tissue which is stained green (solid arrows) and megalocytosis (open arrows). (Stain: Masson's trichrome; magnification, ×40.)

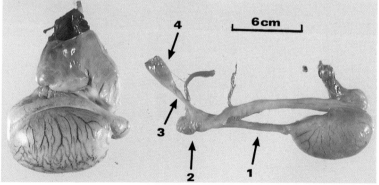

Figure 281

165

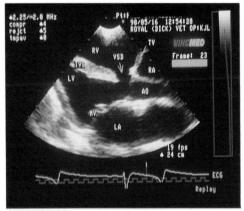

Figure 282

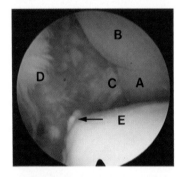

Figure 283. Second carpal bone (A); radial facet of third carpal bone (B); medial dorsal intercarpal ligament (C); synovial membrane (D); dorsodistal articular surface of radial carpal bone (E); chip fracture (arrow).

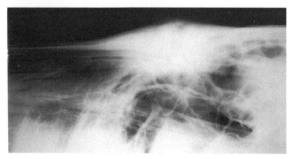

Figure 284

Figure 285

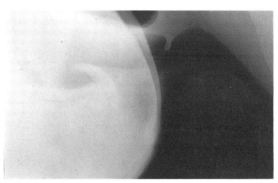

Figure 286

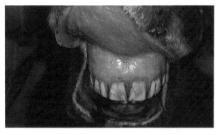

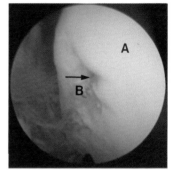

Figure 287. Radial facet of third carpal bone (A); cartilage fibrillation at dorsal margin of lesion (B); entrance to subchondral defect (arrow).

Figure 288. The dorsal band of the caecum (>) leads to the antimesenteric band of the ileum, and its lateral band (>>) is continuous with the free lateral band of the right ventral colon.

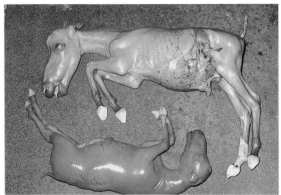

Figure 289A

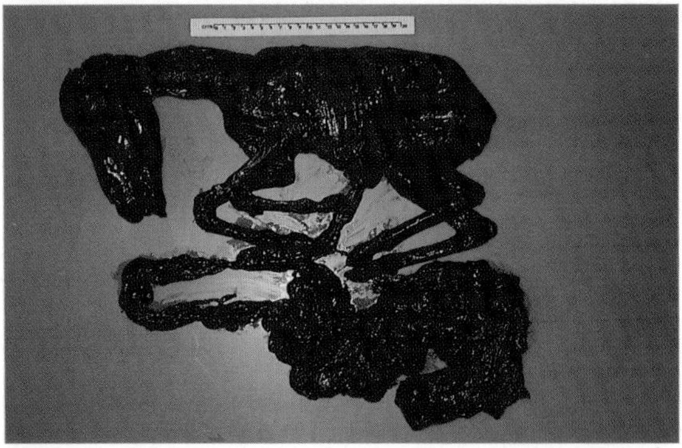

Figure 289B

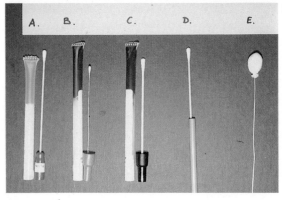

Figure 290

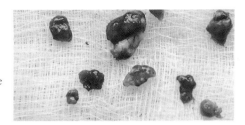

Figure 291. Synovial membrane biopsy samples taken from numerous sites in the femoropatellar joint.

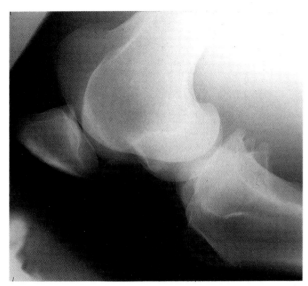

Figure 292

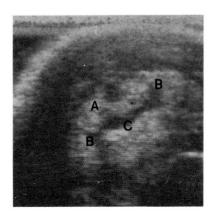

Figure 293 Deep digital flexor tendon (A); Medial and lateral branches of the superficial digital flexor tendon (B); straight sesamoidean ligament (C).

169

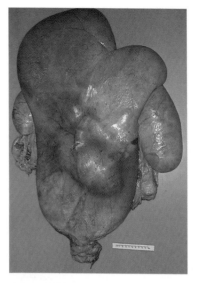

Figure 294A

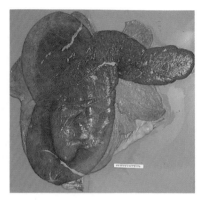

Figure 294B

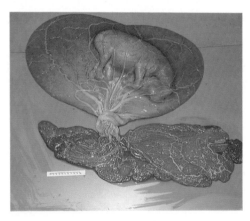

Figure 294C

170

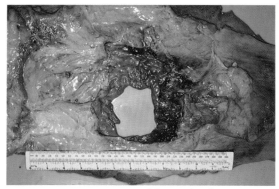

Figure 295. Full-thickness tear of the rectal wall.

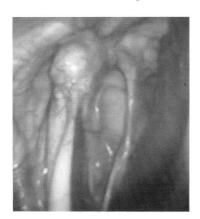

Figure 296

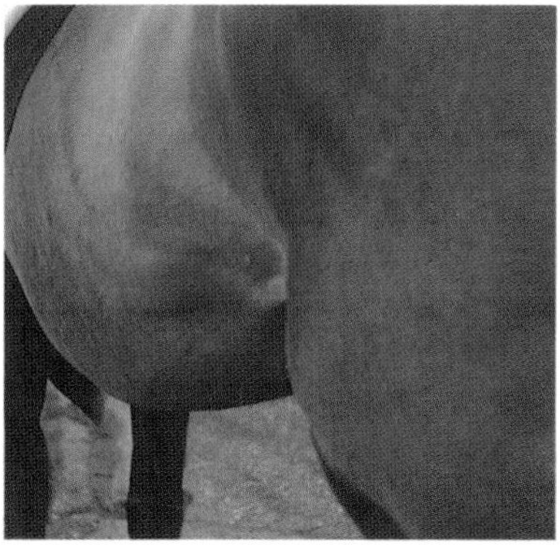

Figure 297A

Figure 297B

171

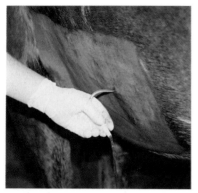

Figure 297C

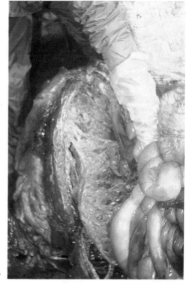

Figure 297D

Figure 298A

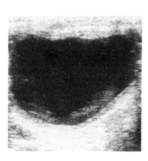

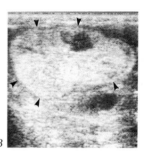

Figure 298B

Figure 298C

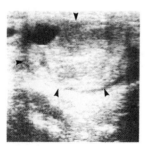

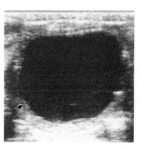

Figure 298D

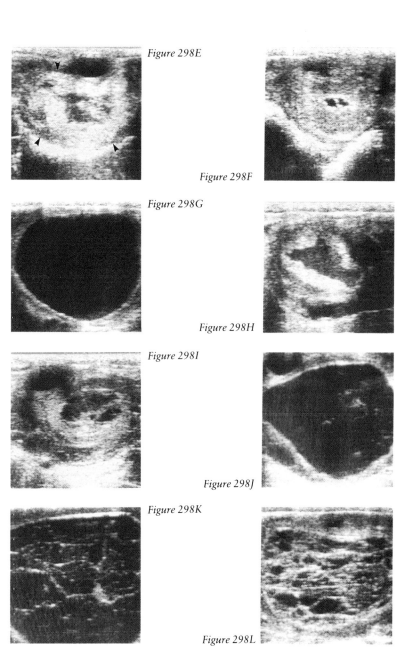

Figure 298E

Figure 298F

Figure 298G

Figure 298H

Figure 298I

Figure 298J

Figure 298K

Figure 298L

173

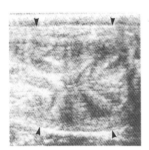

Figure 298M

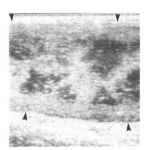

Figure 298N

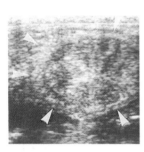

Figure 298O

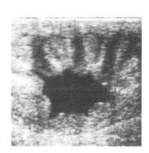

Figure 298P

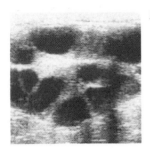

Figure 298Q

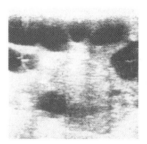

Figure 298R

Figure 299

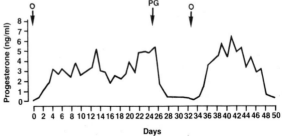

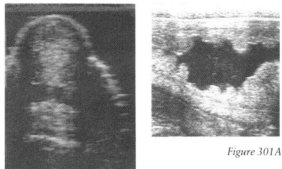

Figure 300

Figure 301A

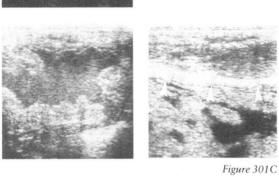

Figure 301B

Figure 301C

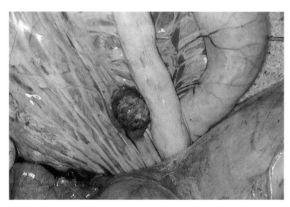

Figure 302A

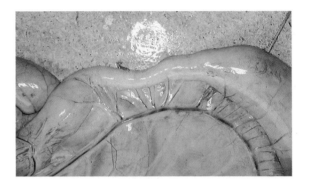

Figure 302B

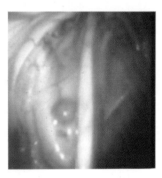

Figure 303

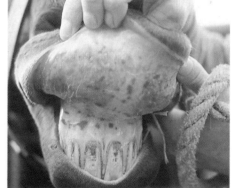

Figure 304

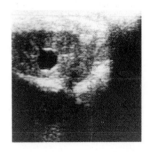

Figure 305A

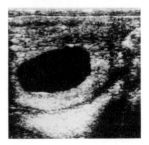

Figure 305B

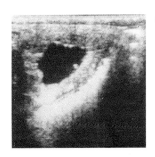

Figure 305C

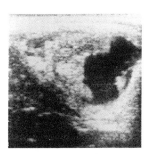

Figure 305D

Figure 305E

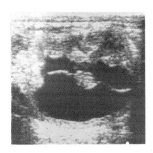

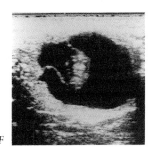

Figure 305F

Figure 305G

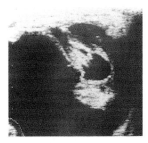

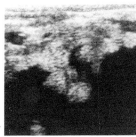

Figure 305H

Figure 305I

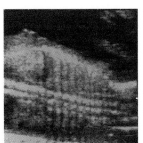

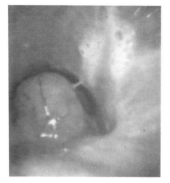

Figure 306A

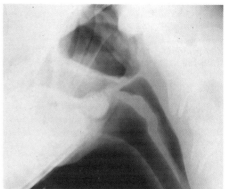

Figure 306B

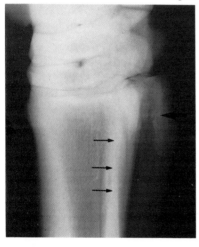

Figure 307

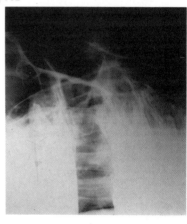

Figure 308

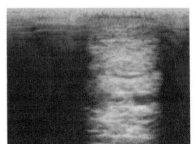

Figure 309

ANSWERS

*Illustrations for the Answers are given in the **Answer Illustrations Section**, pages 159–182.*

1 (a) There is osteochondral fragmentation of the dorsoproximal aspect of the proximal phalanx (*Figure 260*).
(b) The principal differential diagnoses of osteochondral fragmentation of the dorsoproximal articular surface of the proximal phalanx are traumatic chip fractures and osteochondritis dissecans.
(c) The dorsomedial aspect of the joint is most commonly affected.
(d) Localisation of pain by regional analgesia (palmar and palmar metacarpal nerves) or, preferably, intra-articular analgesia. Evaluation of the contralateral limb. Both of the principal differential diagnoses are frequently bilateral.

2 (a) *Figure 2* shows a lateromedial view; other views to obtain are dorsoplantar, dorsolateral–plantaromedial oblique, and plantarolateral–dorsomedial oblique views.
(b) There is an osseous fragment distal to the trochleas of the talus.
(c) The osseous body is probably an osteochondral fragment, a manifestation of osteochondrosis. Such fragments may arise from the distal intermediate ridge of the tibia and fall distally, becoming trapped at the entrance to the talocalcaneal–centroquatral (proximal intertarsal) joint.
(d) In the absence of distension of the tarsocrural (tibiotarsal) joint capsule the fragment is unlikely to be associated with lameness. If the fragment is the cause of lameness, it should be improved by intra-articular analgesia of the tarsocrural joint. Consider blocking the centrodistal (distal intertarsal) and tarsometatarsal joints, remembering that lameness can be associated with a joint without any associated radiographic abnormalities. Such pieces sometimes occur bilaterally, therefore radiographic examination of the contralateral hock may be useful.
(e) The distal end of the lateral trochlea has a large notch.

3 (a) A tracheobronchial foreign body should be suspected. Brambles are the commonest type of such foreign bodies encountered in horses; the thorns act as barbs, allowing distal movement of the bramble, but preventing it from being coughed up. Confirmation of the diagnosis requires the endoscopic visualisation of the foreign body (*Figure 261*).
(b) Removal of the foreign body is frequently not possible in the conscious animal. Endoscopic retrieval under general anaesthesia is usually successful, although the bramble may fragment in the process. A temporary tracheotomy may be required to permit a more direct approach to the lower airways. Treatment with antibiotics is necessary, since the foreign body can induce a bronchitis and/or localised pneumonia.

4 (a) The differential diagnosis includes melanoma, melanosarcoma, and equine sarcoid. Diagnosis is based on the histological evaluation of a biopsy.
(b) For melanoma the prognosis is excellent; for melanosarcoma there is a tendency to metastasise and prognosis is poor to very guarded (may need to amputate the tail); for sarcoid the prognosis should be fair to good but recurrence is not unusual and consideration should be given to concurrent treatment such as cryosurgery, BCG infiltration, etc.

5 (a) This horse is affected by an acute colitis, probably due to acute salmonellosis. Salmonella infection is commonly associated with a stressful condition, such as transportation, recent surgery, or antibiotic therapy. A period of dullness, anorexia, pyrexia, and mild colic often precedes the onset of diarrhoea by up to 4 days.
(b) The diagnosis of salmonellosis depends on the isolation of the organism (from faeces or rectal biopsy). Repeated samples may need to be cultured since the organism is inconsistently shed in the faeces, even in the acute disease. In a small proportion of cases, the isolation of salmonella many only be possible from post-mortem tissues. Haematology often reveals an absolute neutropenia early in the course of the disease, but this is a non-specific sign.
(c) The most important therapeutic consideration is fluid and electrolyte replacement, which frequently requires intensive intravenous fluid therapy. The use of antimicrobial agents in acute salmonellosis is controversial; there is little evidence to suggest that antiobiotic therapy is helpful (unless there is a possibility of septicaemia). Intestinal protectants and absorbents, such as bismuth subsalicylate, activated charcoal, kaolin, and pectin, may provide some minor benefit.

6 (a) Second degree atrioventricular block (Mobitz type II); occasional atrial contraction (electrically signified by a P wave) without subsequent ventricular contraction (QRST complex); constant PR interval. A bifid P wave is also present but this is not considered abnormal in the horse and would not cause an irregularity in pulse rate (*Figure 262*).
(b) Trot the horse up or in some other way excite the animal. Second degree heart block is commonly detected in fit horses and is due to increased vagal tone. In excitement, it generally disappears, and is of no clinical significance in the majority of animals.

7 (a) This was a case of proximal (anterior) enteritis. The main differentiating signs are fever, depression following pain, leucocytosis and peritoneal fluid that has a total protein over 30 g/l with a low WBC count. Gastric reflux is abundant and sometimes orange-brown tinged.
(b) Differentiating proximal (anterior) enteritis from strangulating small intestinal obstruction can be very difficult and a case with these clinical signs should be hospitalised as soon as possible. If there is uncertainty a laparotomy may be necessary (*Figure 263*). Immediate measures should include:
  1. Decompression of the stomach as often as necessary. This also relieves pain.
  2. Rehydration with a balanced electrolyte solution intravenously.
  3. Analgesia, e.g. phenylbutazone or xylazine. Flunixin meglumine is indicated for its antiendotoxic effects in the severe case but one must be aware that it may mask signs of worsening septic shock if the case was in fact a strangulating obstruction.
Treated medically or surgically proximal (anterior) enteritis has a high mortality rate. Close monitoring is essential to differentiate from strangulating bowel disease requiring prompt surgery.

8 (a) The mare has loss of function of the flexor part of the reciprocal apparatus (which normally ensures that the hock flexes when the stifle is flexed). This is due to rupture of the fibularis (peroneus) tertius.
(b) Rupture of the fibularis tertius may result when an animal struggles to free a trapped leg, during exertion at the start of a race, or as a result of falling in a hindlimb cast which maintains the hock in extension.

(c) Unless there has been concurrent injury to the hock, no abnormality will be seen on hock radiographs.

(d) In a small proportion of cases, the loss of function may result from avulsion of the fibularis tertius from its origin in the extensor fossa of the distolateral aspect of the femur. In these cases, a separate fragment of bone may be seen at this site.

9 (a) Probably not.

(b) Auditory tube diverticulum (ATD) (guttural pouch) tympany is the most likely possibility. Bilateral tympany may also be encountered. Most cases are associated with a defect of the ostium (a) of the ATD (guttural pouches). Although no obvious defect is often detectable it is the failure of the ostia to open when deglutition occurs which creates a 'one-way valve' effect. Air allowed into the pouch(es) cannot escape and as there is little restriction to the enlargement laterally the tympanitic swelling develops progressively. Empyema of the ATD should also be considered.

(c) Inspiratory dyspnoea, nasal discharge. Both sides may be affected.

10 (a)
● Early in oestrus the ovaries usually feel irregular due to the presence of several small (+2 cm) follicles. As oestrus progresses one or more follicles grow to attain a size of 3.0–5.0 cm (commonly 3.5–4.0 cm) before ovulation. As follicles mature they become less tense, and can become soft and quite compressible just before ovulation. Oestrus usually terminates 12–48 h after ovulation.
● During the latter part of oestrus the uterus has a compressible, thick-walled texture due to intramural oedema. *Figure 264A* shows the uterine body of a mare in oestrus. The uterus has been incised to reveal the oedematous endometrial folds that are present at this time.
● The cervix is relaxed and oedematous during oestrus; palpably, per rectum, it is soft and indistinct. Fibrosis of the cervix, which occurs in older mares, can make the cervix feel uncharacteristically hard and tight.

(b)
● After ovulation the collapsed follicle refills with blood to form the corpus haemorrhagicum (CH); this is usually a little smaller than the follicle that preceded it, but may be bigger. Initially the texture of the CH may be similar to that of a follicle, with which it may be confused. As the CH becomes organised and invaded with luteal tissue it becomes smaller, firmer in texture, and drawn into the ovary (surrounded by stroma). By the fourth to fifth day after ovulation it is usually no longer palpable. *Figure 264B* shows a 4-day-old CH in a pony ovary; luteal tissue is developing peripherally. During the rest of dioestrus variable degrees of follicular growth may be detected.
● Increasing progesterone dominance causes the now non-oedematous uterus to become smaller and more cylindrical due to contraction of the myometrium. During normal dioestrus the palpable texture of the uterus due to this change is quite variable, but in general, towards the end of the progesterone-dominant period (14 days post ovulation), the uterus is said to have acquired tone (a firm, rubbery texture associated with a tubular shape to the uterine horns).
● Progesterone also causes contraction of the cervix, which occurs progressively during early dioestrus. By 5–7 days after ovulation the cervix is palpably firm, +7 cm in length and +1 cm in diameter (fibrosis in older mares may mimic this textural effect). After the corpus luteum (CL) regresses, gradual relaxation of the cervix occurs.

(c)
- The length of time for which mares have ovarian inactivity in the winter and spring is very variable. If the period of time is short (1–2 months) the ovaries may continue to contain small (palpable) follicles due to continued follicle-stimulating hormone (FSH) release and the mare is then said to be in 'shallow' anoestrus. In more prolonged periods of ovarian quiescence (deep anoestrus) the ovaries feel completely inactive (hard texture, regular bean-like shape with easily palpable ovulation fossa).
- Irrespective of the follicular content of the ovaries in anoestrus the uterus becomes very thin-walled and indistinct (flaccid) and may be difficult to locate on palpation.
- The anoestrus cervix can almost 'disappear' due to lack of hormonal stimulation; it then becomes an easily dilatable 'ring' between the vagina and uterus. Per rectum it is usually soft and difficult to distinguish from the surrounding tissues. The cervices of mares in anoestrus are similar to those in oestrus when palpated per rectum, but are very different when palpated or visualised per vagina.

(d) Prolonged dioestrus occurs commonly in mares because of a failure of luteolysis at the usual time. The palpable features of the tract become more intense, i.e.:
- The ovaries, although they contain a non-palpable CL, become more irregular due to the growth of many follicles to 2.0–2.5 cm diameter; often one follicle may become larger and, occasionally, ovulations occur during prolonged dioestrus.
- Uterine tone may increase, so that after several weeks it may resemble that of early pregnancy.
- The palpable firmness of the cervix also becomes more marked, as in early gestation.

11 (a) The pony is showing excessive salivation and reflux of bile-stained fluid containing food material.
(b) The differential diagnosis should include the following: gastric disorders – primary and secondary gastric dilatation; small intestinal obstruction – e.g. intraluminal obstruction, intramural haematoma or oedema, topographical alterations such as volvulus, herniation through natural or pathological openings or intussusception; caecal disorders – ileocaecal or caecocolic intussusception; functional obstructions – grass sickness, paralytic ileus associated with peritonitis, proximal enteritis or ragwort poisoning. Dysphagia in addition to reflux of bile-stained fluid in a horse with colic is strongly suggestive of acute grass sickness. Excessive salivation is a useful sign as it provides some evidence for dysphagia which may otherwise be difficult to detect on clinical examination of a horse which will not attempt to eat or drink.
(c) Reduced gut sounds, abdominal distension, tachycardia, patchy sweating and fine muscle tremors. The rectum may contain small mucous-coated faecal balls. Firm impaction of the large colon with the corrugated feel typical of secondary impaction occurs. Small intestinal distension is occasionally present.

12 (a) Lateromedial, dorsoproximal–palmarodistal oblique and palmaroproximal–palmarodistal oblique views.
(b) The view in *Figure 9A* is not a true lateromedial projection and exposure is not ideal for evaluation of corticomedullary definition, and structure of the cortex of the navicular bone. Repeated views were no better and yielded no additional information. The view in *Figure 9B* shows at least six variably shaped and sized lucent zones along the distal border of the navicular bone. There is modelling of the proximal border and the lateral margin of the navicular bone. No diagnosis is possible from these radiographs.

(c) There is mineralisation on the flexor cortex of the navicular bone at and slightly medial to the sagittal ridge. Corticomedullary definition is fair and there is no evidence of medullary sclerosis.

(d) *Figure* 9C shows a palmaroproximal–palmarodistal oblique view, which is obtained with the foot to be examined standing on a cassette, caudal to the contralateral foot with the fetlock joint extended. The X-ray machine is positioned beneath the horse's abdomen with the beam centred between the bulbs of the heel, angled at approximately 45° to the horizontal.

(e) Diagnosis is mineralisation on the flexor cortex of the navicular bone; prognosis is poor.

Figure 265 illustrates the boiled-out bony specimen. Histological examination of the removed section confirmed the presence of new bone on the flexor surface.

13 (a)
- Strip the avulsed horn from the coronet. It may be helpful to sedate the mare and to perform palmar (abaxial sesamoid) nerve blocks.
- Place on a bar shoe with side clips to prevent movement of the wall.
- Keep shod until new horn has completely grown down. This is likely to take at least 1 year.

(b) No, provided that there has not been damage to the coronary band *per se*. If there has been excessive damage to the coronary band then subsequent hoof wall growth will be abnormal. Uncomplicated cases respond well to stripping the wall off and to corrective shoeing, provided that there is not excessive laminar damage. The prognosis is good for breeding purposes but would be more guarded for return to athletic function.

(c) Only until the hoof has grown back to ground level.

Table 5. Clinical features of the reproductive tract in prolonged dioestrus and the transition from anoestrus to the breeding season.

	Transition	Prolonged dioestrus
Ovaries		
Palpation	Lobulated	Lobulated
Ultrasound	Many follicles	Many follicles and corpora lutea
Uterus		
Palpation	Doughy or flaccid	Tonic (contracted and tubular)
Ultrasound	Homogeneous or oedematous	Homogeneous
Cervix		
Palpation per rectum	Soft and indistinct	Hard and cylindrical
Palpation per vaginam	Relaxed – vagina may be moist	Constricted, tonic and protruding – vagina dry
Speculum examination	May be slight hyperaemia, oedema and moistness	Dry, pale and protruding into vagina
Progesterone plasma concentration[a]	<1 ng/ml	> 1 ng/ml

[a] This test may be required by inexperienced clinicians.
Note: fibrosis of the cervix in old mares may produce similar palpable features, per rectum, to those in dioestrus.

14 There is no condition in the mare which can really be called 'cystic ovaries' and terms such as 'a touch cystic', etc., are used by those who have little knowledge of the reproductive biology of mares. The term 'cystic' implies the presence and persistence of morphologically abnormal structures which may interfere with the normal reproductive behaviour of the animal; such structures do not occur in the mare.

Conditions which, for one reason or another, may be erroneously referred to as cystic ovaries are:

- Parovarian cysts: small cysts on the surface of the ovary, the mesosalpinx or the fimbria. They are remnants of the Wolffian ducts and are extremely rarely thought to interfere with fertility. Most are less than 1.5 cm diameter but may be palpated or detected on ultrasound scan.
- Persistent follicles due to seasonal influence. During the transition from anoestrus to cyclic behaviour there is often a prolonged period (up to 2 months or more) when follicles are stimulated to grow in the ovaries but do not become mature enough to ovulate. Palpably and ultrasonographically the ovaries contain many follicles 2 cm in diameter and feel lobular. Since sequential examinations reveal a similar appearance (even though some follicles will have become atretic and replaced by others) in the ovaries, it may be assumed that the apparent static nature of the ovaries has occurred due to an inherent lesion. However, the ovaries are not producing ovulatory follicles because of insufficient pituitary activity – all the follicles in the ovaries are normal but in an arrested state of development. None have an abnormal histological appearance and they are not cysts.
- Prolonged dioestrus. Persistence of the corpus luteum for 3 months or more is relatively common in the mare; it occurs after a normal oestrus and ovulation and is caused by a fault in the luteolytic mechanism in mares that both have or have not been mated. The development of small follicles (<2 cm) is common during normal dioestrus although occasionally larger ones are found. As prolonged dioestrus proceeds, progressively more follicles of 2–4 cm develop and the ovaries become irregular and lobulated and can feel 'cystic'. The condition can occur at any time of year, and features which distinguish it from those of the seasonal transition are shown in *Table 5*.
- Granulosa cell tumours have pathological 'cystic' cavities and are discussed in Question 95, as are two very rare conditions which do not interfere with the normal cyclic activity of the other ovary.
- Very small (2–5 mm) cysts have occasionally been found in the area of the ovulation fossa of old mares; they are thought to be formed by pieces of the fimbriae which have been drawn into the ovary by developing corpora haemorrhagica. It is possible that when they are present in large numbers they could physically interfere with ovulation. They are not palpable per rectum and have not been characterised ultrasonographically.

15 (a) The differential diagnosis of scrotal swelling in a gelding includes: scirrhous cord, suture abscess, oedema, cystic ends (inguinal hernia in the gelding unassociated with the immediate castration procedure is extremely rare).
(b) Scirrhous cord – a botryomycotic lesion associated with a low grade staphylococcal infection, resulting in microabscessation and extensive fibrous tissue development.
(c) Hindlimb lameness, muscle atrophy, enlarged inguinal lymph nodes (palpated per rectum), neutrophilia with a left shift, increased total plasma protein and fibrinogen concentrations.

(d) Careful dissection and radical surgical excision of the diseased fibrous tissue. This procedure should be preceded by a 10-day course of antibiotics in an attempt to reduce the lesion size. Postoperative management involves daily irrigation of the wound, which is allowed to heal by secondary intention.

(e) The prognosis is dependent on the complete resection of diseased tissue before the ascending infection involves the abdominal cavity.

16 (a) Progressive ethmoidal haematoma.
- Coagulopathies associated with warfarin treatment or other causes such as chronic hepatic failure, specific clotting factor deficiencies or thrombocytopenia.
- Nasal polyps, nasal varicosity.
- Erosions of blood vessels within the ipsilateral auditory tube diverticulum (ATD) (guttural pouch).

(b)
- Accurate assessment of clotting mechanisms including an assessment of platelet function.
- Radiography (lateral and dorsoventral or ventrodorsal views).
- Endoscopy.

The primary objective is to establish the site of the blood loss and thereby establish the possible causes. Haemorrhagic diatheses are rare in the horse and would probably be associated with other sites of bleeding, but in this case administration of warfarin might have been involved. Radiographically ethmoidal haematoma may be seen as a clearly defined radiopaque lesion visible in lateral and ventrodorsal projections rostral to the ethmoid turbinate bone. Endoscopically the lesions generally appear as well-defined yellow-green or dark masses in the caudal nasal cavity. The lesions may be small but are commonly extensive and may progress to considerable size when both nostrils may become involved. Serious dyspnoea may arise. ATD (guttural pouch) mycosis and nasal polyps, nasal varicosity and other small bleeding foci may be identified positively by endoscopy. Angiography may be useful in the assessment of ATD mycosis.

17 (a) The clinical signs and history are highly suggestive of larval cyathostomiasis. Larval stages of the small strongyles (cyathostomes) are capable of encysting within the mucosa of the caecum and colon, where they can remain in large numbers for long periods of time; in this state they appear to be protected from the action of routine anthelmintics. Under certain circumstances the larvae may emerge en masse, causing damage to the mucosa and stimulating a severe inflammatory reaction which results in diarrhoea and protein-losing enteropathy. The disease most commonly affects young adult horses during the winter and spring, and the problem sometimes occurs several days after the routine use of anthelmintics.

Rectal examination and gentle scraping of the mucosa frequently reveal numerous cyathostome larvae. Since the disease is associated with strongyle larvae, the faecal worm egg count may be zero. Haematological changes are non-specific. Biochemical evaluation often shows hypoalbuminaemia and elevation of β_1-globulins. Precise confirmation of the diagnosis is only possible by bowel wall biopsy, but the above findings are generally considered satisfactory to make the diagnosis. The isolation of salmonellae is unlikely to be of clinical significance in this case, and requires no specific treatment, although hygiene measures should be instituted to prevent the spread of the organism to other horses or to humans. When the primary condition resolves, the shedding of salmonellae will probably cease.

(b) Therapy should involve repeated use of larvicidal anthelmintics (e.g. ivermectin 200 µg/kg or fenbendazole 30 mg/kg); the possibility of benzimidazole resistance of the cyathostomes should be considered. Concomitant therapy with corticosteroids to control the mucosal inflammation is often helpful. Fluid and electrolyte therapy is sometimes necessary if the animal is severely dehydrated.

18 (a) The clinical means of assessing intestinal viability include:
- Colour and appearance of the intestinal wall.
- Colour of the mesentery and pulsation of mesenteric vessels.
- The presence of gut motility.
- The colour and appearance of the mucosa as inspected via an enterotomy incision.

The need for resection is indicated by:
- Discoloured, thickened or oedematous bowel and the failure of the normal pink colour of the bowel wall to return after correction of the strangulating lesion (*Figure 266A*).
- Haemorrhage and thrombosis of the mesenteric vessels (*Figure 266A*).
- Failure of normal peristalsis to return and the appearance of enlarged empty, flaccid, hose-pipe-like loops of bowel after decompression.
- Dark reddened or blackish mucosa that indicates sloughing, and the absence of bleeding from the enterotomy incision.

Because clinical assessment based on these criteria is not uniformly reliable, alternative techniques for intraoperative use in the horse (intravenous sodium fluorescein, Doppler measurements of intramural flow) are presently under investigation.

In equivocal cases the surgeon should not hesitate to resect some normal bowel rather than risk leaving compromised bowel in place.

(b) In surgical practice both techniques have their supporters and problems are seldom related to the technique used. The end-to-end technique is technically easier to perform and less time consuming. The side-to-side technique allows selection of a larger stoma, but pocketing of ingesta in the blind pouch of the anastomosis can lead to stasis and necrosis.

(c)
- Everting suture patterns (*Figure 266B*) are not acceptable since the everted mucosa forms a nidus for inflammation, infection, abscessation, adhesions and peritonitis.
- Opposing sutures (*Figure 266C*) theoretically provide the best alignment and produce rapid primary healing. However, they increase the potential for adhesions up to 50%.
- Inverting sutures (*Figure 266D*) produce less adhesions but healing is delayed because of poor anatomical alignment. Bowel wall inversion can compromise intraluminal diameter and result in stenosis. In practice these considerations do not seem to be a problem.
- A double-layer closure composed of an opposing inner layer and an inverting outer seromuscular layer (*Figure 266E*) is strong, can be adequately sealed and produces minimal adhesions. Because only one layer is inverted, reduction of luminal diameter is minimal.

The use of inverting or double-layer closure techniques is advisable in intestinal anastomosis in the horse.

(d)
- Synthetic multifilament absorbable suture materials (polyglycolic acid and polyglactin 910) are commonly used for intestinal closure in the horse.

- Chromic catgut produces an undesirable cellular inflammatory response and is subject to proteolytic breakdown.
- Monofilament materials have no capillarity but are more difficult to handle as they kink.

(e) The mucosal eversion obtained with this technique results in extensive adhesion and stricture formation associated with postoperative colic.

19 (a) The murmur is indicative of tricuspid regurgitation. The colour flow study shows a jet of blood in the right atrium during systole.

(b) The murmur was an incidental finding, and the horse is continuing to perform well. The murmur was only audible in a localised area. The colour flow map reveals a narrow jet in a localised area of the right atrium close to the tricuspid valve. The tricuspid valve does not appear to be thickened. All of these factors indicate that the murmur is of limited significance; however, further information is required. The resting heart rate of the horse should be known. The appearance of the jugular veins and the degree of jugular pulsation would give an indication of the right atrial pressure. The response of the heart to exercise should be determined. It would be helpful to see the videotape of the ultrasound study in order to obtain a clear view of the tricuspid valve and its movement. An assessment of the right ventricular size should be made and a Doppler study to determine the velocity of the regurgitant jet would be helpful as this would give an indication of the pressure gradient between the right ventricle and right atrium.

(c) Mild tricuspid regurgitation is unlikely to affect this animal's performance as a dressage horse. There is little data available on the progression of this condition, although it is known that some horses continue to perform well with no deterioration in valve function. There is no evidence of valve thickening in this case, which would indicate a progressive condition.

20 (a) Peritonitis. Rupture of the gastrointestinal tract is a common cause of peritonitis but few horses survive more than a few hours. A very careful search should be made for other causes which include intestinal infarction following thromboembolism of mesenteric arteries, strangulating obstruction of the intestine (unlikely in chronic cases), intestinal penetration by a foreign body, abscessation, injury to the reproductive tract, and systemic disease.

(b) Peritoneal fluid analysis is the only reliable diagnostic parameter for peritonitis. Even this may be difficult to obtain if the lesion is walled off. Peritoneal fluid smears should be examined for bacteria and a bacteriological culture performed. Persistent pyrexia and parietal pain (manifest by abdominal guarding) are two more useful clinical signs, and the rectum feels as though it is partially held by surrounding tissues in some cases. A wide variety of clinical signs may be seen, including weight loss, diarrhoea and even gastric reflux. Ultrasonography or laparoscopy may be useful diagnostic procedures.

(c)
- Antibiotics. Large doses for long periods (7 days to 1 month) of broad-spectrum antibiotics are essential, e.g. trimethoprim/sulphadioxine and penicillin in combination.
- Non-steroidal anti-inflammatories and analgesics such as phenylbutazone or flunixin meglumine.
- Intravenous fluid therapy should be given if necessary.
- Peritoneal lavage occasionally helps but is often unrewarding and stressful to the animal.

- Anthelmintics will be appropriate in cases thought to have verminous involvement.
- Laparotomy may be necessary if there is an intestinal obstruction or a palpable lesion that may be operable.

21 (a) *Culicoides* hypersensitivity, *Oxyuris* infestation or psoroptic mange mites.
(b) Squamous cell carcinoma of the vulva lip and clitoris.
(c) Total ablation of the clitoris was successful, with no recurrence over 5 years.

22 Sample A appears to be clear, normal-coloured synovial fluid with streaks of bright fresh blood. This is indicative of iatrogenic haemorrhage during collection. Sample B is xanthochromic, opaque, and has a proteinaceous froth at the surface. This is highly indicative of synovial sepsis.

The joint from which sample A was obtained requires no further attention *per se*. Case B should receive urgent treatment if a functional joint is to be maintained. This may include lavage, arthroscopic debridement and lavage or arthrotomy and lavage, combined with aggressive systemic antimicrobial therapy. The use of intra-articular antimicrobials is currently considered unjustified by the majority although recent evidence supports their use. The results of laboratory determinations (principally cytology, protein concentration and bacteriological investigations) are of assistance in case management but should not delay treatment.

23 (a) Dorsoplantar, lateromedial, dorsolateral–plantaromedial oblique and plantarolateral–dorsomedial oblique views.
(b) A lateromedial view is seen in *Figure 19A*. There is a suggestion of large osteophyte formation on the dorsoproximal aspect of the third metatarsal bone with an horizontal lucent line traversing it. The third tarsal bone appears to narrow in a proximodistal direction approximately 1 cm plantar to its dorsal aspect. A plantarolateral–dorsomedial oblique view is seen in *Figure 19B*. The above observations are confirmed.
(c) A dorsolateral–plantaromedial oblique (D 80°L-PIMO) view should help to isolate the osteophyte formation (*Figure 267*).
(d) Intra-articular analgesia of the tarsometatarsal joint. Lameness was very substantially improved.
(e) It is likely that osteophyte formation developed secondarily to malformation of the third tarsal bone. The latter may have been due to incomplete ossification of the bone at birth and its subsequent compression or possibly osteochondrosis.

24 (a)
- Discharge from the vulva, especially at the end of dioestrus and 24 h after covering.
- Conformation suggesting pneumovagina.
- Hearing the mare aspirate air into the vagina.
- Seeing exudate in the vagina during speculum examination; if it is frothy, suspect pneumovagina.
- Short oestrus cycles suggest endometritis; inflammation appears to stimulate premature release of prostaglandin by the uterus and early regression of the corpus luteum (CL) (*Figure 268*). Whether or not this is reflected in an overall reduction of cycle length (19 or less days) depends on the length of the follicular phase. However, a return to oestrus less than 16 days after the end of the previous oestrus suggests a short luteal phase. Mares with severe endometrial damage and chronic endometritis may have long cycles (i.e. persistent CLs).

188

- If routine testing for endometritis is not carried out, failure of a mare to conceive to coverings at two successive oestrus periods by a fertile stallion warrants investigation.

(b) Palpation of the uterus may reveal the presence of a large volume of exudate; chronic accumulation of pus occurs usually because there is a cervical lesion (adhesions or stenosis) which prevents or severely restricts escape of the pus. Affected mares usually cycle normally or have short cycles, especially in the early stages.

- Ultrasonography of the uterus may reveal fluid in the lumen. In early oestrus small amounts of fluid are probably normal but may indicate that the mare may experience problems expelling fluids after mating. Larger amounts of cloudy fluid, especially after mating and during the luteal phase, indicate that endometritis is probable. Care should be taken to distinguish fluid in the uterine lumen from urine in the bladder; the latter can have a very variable appearance being either totally clear (black), full of calcium salts (white) or demarcated into patterns involving both the above.
- Intrauterine swab sampling. A guarded method is recommended to prevent contamination of the swab. After collection it should be plated out for routine culture (blood and MacConkey's agar), and may be also for microaerophilic organisms (*Taylorella equigenitalis*) and anaerobes. A smear should also be made on a microscope slide and stained by any method used for blood smears; the presence of neutrophils suggests endometritis and the presence of endometrial (cuboidal or columner) epithelial cells confirms that an endometrial sample was obtained.
- Endometrial biopsy. Inflammatory cells in the tissues denote inflammation. Neutrophils suggest acute inflammation and lymphocytes and eosinophils suggest 'chronic' conditions.

(c)
- In cases where pneumovagina is a problem, Caslick's or Pouret's operations should be used.
- To prevent uterine contamination during mating, artificial insemination (AI) can be used in non-Thoroughbred mares. Extending the semen in a diluent which contains antibiotics should reduce bacterial growth significantly but is not always totally successful. In Thoroughbreds, where AI is not permitted, the minimal contamination technique has been used: a 200-ml volume of semen extender, including antibiotics, is placed into the uterus immediately before natural mating. The ejaculate then meets the antibiotic medium and, theoretically, bacterial growth is suppressed. The results of this technique are equivocal. After foaling, contamination of the involuting uterus has been reduced by suturing the vulva or placing metal (Michel) clips across the dorsal orifice.

(d) So many methods are used to treat endometritis that only a few general principle's can be discussed.
- Where chronic endometritis is established in barren mares, repeated saline irrigations using a Foley catheter may be necessary to remove inspissated pus, followed by antibiotic treatment.
- Post-partum endometritis is usually associated with retained placenta. Irrigation of saline (introduction and subsequent siphonage) should be carried out at least once a day followed by intrauterine instillation of antibiotics.
- Most efforts are directed towards preventing bacteria, which are inevitably introduced during mating, from establishing in the uterus. Treatments are therefore carried out after mating, and uterine interferences can be safely employed for 3 days after ovulation (the fertilised ovum doesn't reach the uterus until the fifth day). This involves the instillation of antibiotics into the uterus after covering. Because there is

no time to collect samples for identification of bacteria and antibiotic sensitivity testing, broad-spectrum combinations are usually used. These include penicillin (for streptococci) and antimicrobials likely to kill Gram-negative organisms and anaerobes (streptomycin, neomycin, framycetin, nitrofurantoin, gentamicin and polymyxin).

The dose and volume of vehicle (saline or water) employed varies greatly, but in general it is worth noting that small volumes do penetrate the lumen well and large volumes may stimulate reflux per vaginam.

Non-antibiotic substances, e.g. dilute antiseptics, hydrogen peroxide, etc., have also been used to treat bacterial endometritis.

25 (a) Control of the seizures (using diazepam, phenobarbital, phenytoin, or a combination of these drugs) is the most immediate concern. Other important considerations are to protect the foal from self-induced trauma, particularly to the eyes, provide oxygen supplementation, reduce body temperature (alcohol, cold water, fans, and possibly antipyretics).

(b) Complete blood count and fibrinogen (to address the possibility of sepsis-related seizures), blood glucose, electrolytes (sodium, potassium, calcium, chloride and bicarbonate, including total CO_2) and IgG determination.

(c) Neonatal maladjustment syndrome, trauma, infection, electrolyte abnormalities, congenital malformation, liver failure, heat stroke.

(d) Good (>80%) for complete recovery (no residual deficits) from neonatal maladjustment syndrome, providing IgG levels are good, seizures are controlled promptly, and around-the-clock nursing care is available for the first few days of life.

26 (a) No, optic atrophy can be seen.

(b) Pale optic disc with absence of blood vessels, together with areas of retinal degeneration.

27 (a) Lateromedial, dorsoproximal–palmarodistal oblique and palmaroproximal–palmarodistal oblique views.

(b) There are at least seven variably shaped and sized lucent zones along the distal border of the navicular bone. There is slight modelling of the proximal border of the bone.

(c) There is considerable controversy surrounding the interpretation of radiographs of the navicular bone, especially of such lucent zones. It is generally accepted that up to seven lucent zones may be within the normal variation, depending to an extent on their size and shape. An increase in number and/or size of these lucent zones, synovial invaginations, may reflect the bone's vascular response accompanying adaptive modelling, which occurs in both sound and lame horses. Additional information should be obtained from the lateromedial and palmaroproximal–palmarodistal oblique views, which were within the normal range. It may also be useful to radiograph the contralateral foot (which was similar in appearance). These radiographic findings are considered to be of unlikely clinical significance.

Lameness associated with navicular disease is usually, but not invariably, improved (or eliminated) by perineural analgesia of the palmar digital nerves, and alleviated by palmar (abaxial sesamoid) nerve blocks. The pattern of lameness in this horse is not typical of navicular disease.

(d)
- Ultrasonographic examination of the palmar soft tissues of the pastern region. (The deep digital flexor tendon was enlarged but of normal echogenicity in this area.)
- Intra-articular analgesia of the distal interphalangeal joint. (Negative.)
- Analgesia of the navicular bursa. (Negative.)

Post-mortem examination confirmed a diagnosis of strain of the deep digital flexor tendon (*Figure 269*).

28 (a) If this animal's lameness has not responded to palmar digital nerve blocks, it is probably not suffering from conditions which would cause palmar foot pain such as navicular disease, navicular fractures, a wing fracture of the distal phalanx, or corns. It is also possible that the animal has only partially responded to a palmar digital nerve block. If this is the case, it may still have navicular disease as not all cases of navicular disease respond totally to palmar digital nerve blocks. Alternatively, the animal may have a combination of navicular disease and some other cause of lameness.
(b) The palmar nerves are being blocked at the level of the proximal sesamoid bones. This is known as an abaxial sesamoid nerve block.
(c) The clinician is likely to either perform a four-point block, blocking the palmar nerves and the palmar metacarpal nerves above the level of the fetlock, or intra-articular analgesia of the metacarpophalangeal (fetlock) joint. There is no point in proceeding to try to image a lesion until the site of pain has been established!

29 (a) Ptosis, catarrhal/purulent ocular discharge, drooping of the left ear and flaccidity of the left muzzle and ipsilateral lip.
(b) Facial paralysis.
(c) The duration of the signs and the presence/absence of complicating factors such as damage to the cranial sympathetic trunk. Complete disruption of the nerve may result in permanent changes but local bruising and inflammation may subside with a return to normal function.

30 (a) The differential diagnosis included chronic infection of the upper airway and its associated lymph nodes, and neoplasia. The clinical features are typical of the multicentric form of lymphosarcoma. Chronic infections rarely result in nodular swellings of the pharyngeal/laryngeal mucosa; in contrast, these are relatively common in cases of multicentric lymphosarcoma.
(b) Haematological examination may not aid the differentiation between infective and neoplastic disorders; leucocytosis, neutrophilia and hyperfibrinogenaemia are common in both diseases. Confirmation of the diagnosis will depend on the biopsy of an enlarged lymph node and/or mucosal mass.

31 (a)
- Debride devitalised tissue and thoroughly lavage the wound.
- Dress the leg until a granulation tissue bed is established.
- Cut granulation back to form a uniform bed 2–4 mm deep.
- Medicate for 2–3 days with povidone iodine-soaked bandages to reduce bacterial contamination to a very low level.
- Apply a skin graft.
(b) Occasionally, donor sites produce white hairs or white spots.
- Use donor site from under the mane (with the owner's permission).
- Use belly skin, but remember hair will grow excessively long on grafts from this area.

32 (a) Nephrosplenic entrapment (left dorsal displacement) of the large colon.
(b) Midline laparotomy and surgical relocation of the displaced left colon. If excessive distension or impaction of the colon is present, the left dorsal and ventral colons are evacuated prior to any reduction.
(c) An alternative treatment without laparotomy has been developed. The horse is placed on its back with the hindlimbs raised in hobbles by a hoist. This causes the large colon to fall forward. The horse is then lowered onto its left side and rotated manually onto its sternum and then over to its right side. This procedure offers a significantly high chance of spontaneous resolution.
(d) The prognosis is good providing correction is undertaken promptly. Localised damage to the bowel wall and adhesion formation are rare complications. Recurrence has not been reported.
(e) Displacement of the spleen ventrally and subsequent engorgement may result in direct accidental puncture of the spleen, producing Frank blood.

33 (a) The requirement for protein was originally thought to show little or no increase with exercise. However, sweat contains around 1–1.5 g nitrogen/kg and an apparent increase in nitrogen retention has been shown in working horses. It may therefore be preferable to calculate protein requirements per energy unit fed. This means that with the increasing intake needed to meet energy demands the proportional increase in protein intake will meet requirements. For younger animals there is an increased requirement for protein for growth. This has led the National Research Council, 1989, to recommend the following:

- 40 g crude protein (CP)/Mcal of digestible energy (DE) (5 g digestible crude protein (DCP)/MJ of DE) for maintenance and for exercise.
- 50 g CP/Mcal of DE for weanlings.
- 45 g CP/Mcal of DE for yearlings.

(b) There is some controversy over the effect of too much protein, with some workers suggesting no detrimental *or* beneficial effects on performance, whilst others suggest that effects such as early fatigue in endurance horses may occur. It has been suggested that the intake of more than 2 g DCP/kg body weight/day should be avoided because of the possible effects on water intake, plasma urea and ammonia levels. High protein levels may also affect renal phosphorus and calcium losses although this has been disputed.
(c) The *quality* and nature of the protein in the feedstuffs is very important, especially in the growing horse. The site of protein absorption is also important. (Proteins digested in the small intestine are more likely to be absorbed as amino acids whereas proteins reaching the large intestine are likely to result in ammonia absorption.) Protein digestibility also varies not only with the source of the protein but also the concentration in the diet and possibly exercise, e.g. increasing the concentrate to hay ratio to 1 : 1 can cause an increase in protein digestibility but very high ratios may in fact reduce digestibility. Light exercise, or perhaps improved conditioning as the result of such exercise, may increase protein digestibility. Horses are one of the few domestic animals for which dietary amino acid requirements have not been established. Much of the work has concentrated on lysine which has been shown to be the most limiting amino acid in typical horse diets. Cereals tend to have a relatively poor amino acid profile; and levels of 2.1, 1.9, and 1.7 g/Mcal of DE/day for weanlings, yearlings and two year olds have been recommended (NRC, 1989). Threonine may be the second limiting amino acid for yearling horses primarily on forage-based rearing systems. The feeding of relatively small amounts (around 250 g for example) of full fat soya flakes may help to increase

the protein *quality* without markedly increasing the *quantity* of protein fed.

(d) Alternative sources of non-protein nitrogen such as urea have been evaluated recently but highly fermentable dietary fibre seems to be required for efficient utilisation of such high levels of protein replacement and this feeding practice is therefore not thought to be suitable for performance horses. It is also not recommended for growing horses.

34 (a) There is a well-defined, circular radiopaque lesion in the dorsocaudal lung field. This is probably a pulmonary abscess or localised area of pneumonia. Malodorous discharges are usually indicative of anaerobic bacterial infections, which are commonly involved in pneumonia/lung abscesses.

(b) Comparison of right and left lateral radiographs of the chest may be used to confirm the side of the pulmonary lesion; this is probably on the right-hand side (based on the endoscopic findings). The most important diagnostic procedure will be bacteriological culture to aid the choice of appropriate antibiotic therapy. A sample of lower airway discharge should be obtained aseptically for this purpose; this can be achieved by performing a transtracheal aspiration. Cultures should be performed under both aerobic and anaerobic conditions.

35 (a) Acquired indirect inguinal hernia/eventration—prolapse of bowel through the vaginal ring into the scrotum. The bowel has become obstructed, distended and possibly strangulated.

(b) Treat abdominal pain and developing hypovolaemic shock. Minimise the trauma to the herniated intestinal loop and ensure its early return to the abdomen. The bowel may be traumatised as a result of drying, by contamination from the external environment or mechanically. The intestine should be cleansed with warm sterile saline, decompressed and replaced through the deep inguinal ring. A midline coeliotomy may be required to assist in returning the bowel to the abdomen, to assess its viability and to allow a resection and anastamosis procedure to be performed. The superficial inguinal ring should be closed.

(c) A thorough preoperative clinical examination of the inguinal canal has been performed to detect the presence of pre-existing inguinal hernia. Performing the castration using a closed technique would have prevented this condition.

36 (a) Raised ulcerative lesions on the lips may be associated with the development of larvae of *Gasterophilus* spp. flies. Mature larvae are present in the stomach of horses over winter months.

(b) Bots seldom cause any pathological problems even though there may be high numbers. Local oral irritation may cause some inappetence but the lesions are generally of little significance.

37 (a) This horse has a tracheal deformity which is probably congenital or developmental in nature. These lesions may exist for a considerable period of time before the onset of clinical signs; the initiation of clinical signs in this horse probably related to the start of strenuous exercise, which results in increased respiratory effort, thereby exacerbating the effects of airway obstruction. Alternatively, the lesion might have been the result of an unrecognised traumatic insult. Direct chest trauma, especially at maximal inspiration and with a closed glottis, can exert large retractive forces on the intrathoracic trachea which can result in complete or partial rupture. Tracheal stenosis can also occur after surgical tracheostomy, but the site would be expected to be in the more proximal trachea.

(b) Surgical stabilisation of the stenotic area of trachea may be possible (using a prosthesis), but the prognosis for return to athletic potential would be very poor.

38 (a) Eggs of the common bot, *Gasterophilus intestinalis*, which are laid by adult bot flies during the summer months.
(b) Adult bot flies are a cause of annoyance to horses whilst they are depositing eggs on the hairs of the bodycoat, although the flies neither bite nor sting.
The migration of bots to the stomach starts with the horse rubbing and licking the eggs and periodontal ulcerations occur when the first and second larval stages burrow into the oral mucosa, usually around the cheek teeth. These oral lesions do not usually cause clinical signs.
Second and third stage larvae attached to the gastric lining may cause erosive ulcerative lesions but even when very large burdens are present it is unusual for bot larvae to result in clinical signs.
(c) Eggs can be removed from the hairs by clipping or shaving and grooming. Sponging with warm water helps to remove eggs and stimulates artificial hatching of the eggs, rendering them non-infective to the host.
During winter months almost the entire bot population exists within the host stomach. Administration of boticidal drugs is recommended about 1 month after the first winter frosts (which kill adult bot flies). In the UK two drugs are commercially available with boticidal activity, namely dichlorvos and ivermectin. Of the two compounds ivermectin is generally preferred because it has a better activity against other parasite species; dichlorvos is produced for in-feed medication but is not very palatable to many horses.

39 (a)
- Papilloma.
- Squamous cell carcinoma.
- Mixed sarcoid.
(b)
- Papilloma—may be biopsied.
- Squamous cell carcinoma—total excisional biopsy.
- Biopsy is not recommended if certainty of clinical indicators point to a sarcoid.

Since this is a white non-pigmented area and the horse is a Clydesdale, a squamous cell carcinoma is the most likely diagnosis.

40 These signs indicate that the ovary is tender; this occurs most commonly during the 24 h after ovulation. However, some preovulatory follicles also appear to be tender, and occasionally pain may be envinced for more than 24 h after follicular rupture. Rarely, some mares may appear to have tender ovaries at any stage of the cycle.

41 (a) A nasal tube attached to a rope halter, to prevent respiratory obstruction. Alternatively, it could be a stomach tube, but this is unlikely given the exterior length of the tube. A rope halter is much preferable to a head collar with unprotected buckles if one has to be worn by the horse in recovery. Focal pressure from unprotected buckles can result in facial nerve paralysis, as well as in contusions.

(b)
- Nasal congestion often occurs in horses maintained in dorsal recumbency, due to either partial jugular occlusion or the head being a dependent part with respect to the heart.
- Displacement of the soft palate by the oroendotracheal tube during anaesthesia, resulting in respiratory obstruction once the tube is removed.

42 (a) Osteochondritis dissecans.
(b) Removal of the affected cartilage and mineralised tissue until the affected area is bounded by a healthy osteochondral margin. Debridement of the underlying subchondral bone until grossly normal cancellous bone is obtained.
(c) The area of dystrophic endochondral ossification is considered unviable. Healing of the osteochondral defect (in as much as this can occur) takes place principally from unaffected cancellous bone but there may be some contribution from the cartilage margins.

43 (a) The left eye is more prominent than the right (exophthalmos). The third eyelid is more obvious than normal and there is slight swelling proximal to the eye.
(b) Space-occupying lesions such as a retrobulbar abscess, a tear gland adenoma, a pituitary tumour, a squamous cell carcinoma, etc. may be responsible for exophthalmos.
(c) Radiographic examination may identify some radiopaque lesions. Ultrasonography may be used to identify a soft tissue mass and facilitate its biopsy. Aspiration/needle biopsy of suspected abscesses and other masses may also be helpful.

44 (a) The dorsolateral–palmaromedial oblique view is shown. Dorsomedial–palmarolateral oblique, dorsopalmar and flexed lateromedial views should also be obtained.
(b) There is an osseous cyst-like lesion in the distal aspect of the ulnar carpal bone. There is no detectable communication between it and the middle carpal joint. Note also the oval lucent area in the distal radial epiphysis representing an area of incomplete fusion between the lateral styloid process and the distal radial epiphysis.
(c)
- Obtain radiographs of the contralateral limb: osseous cyst-like lesions are often present bilaterally and if seen in association with a unilateral lameness are probably a 'red herring'.
- Perform perineural analgesia of the median and ulnar nerves: lameness associated with an osseous cyst-like lesion should be improved by regional analgesia of the carpal region; intra-articular analgesia is unlikely to be as effective.
- Review the signalment and clinical signs which are suggestive of another problem (see Question 320).
- Perform intra-articular analgesia of the shoulder and elbow joints.

45 (a) Tru-cut biopsy needle (Travenol).
(b) A line is drawn from the point of the shoulder to the tuber coxae on the right side. The site is located where the line crosses the fourteenth intercostal space. The tenth or eleventh space can also be used, especially if the liver is shrunken.
(c) Haemorrhage is a possible complication and prothrombin time, thrombocyte count and whole blood clotting time should be assessed prior to proceeding with the biopsy. Tetanus vaccination status should be checked.

46 (a) Most cases of endometritis are caused by opportunist pathogens which normally inhabit the caudal female tract and the surface of the male genitalia. During mating the bacterial flora of both sites is carried into the anterior vagina and enters the uterus with the ejaculate.

After all matings there is a rapid inflammatory reaction in the endometrium which in genitally healthy mares ensures elimination of bacteria within 24 h or so. In some mares however this infection persists; from amongst the many bacterial species potentially introduced into the uterus, it is usually β-haemolytic streptococci (almost always *Str. zooepidemicus*) and less commonly coliforms. Staphylococci and other streptococci are sometimes isolated concurrently with β-haemolytic streptococci and *E. coli* but rarely in pure culture. The incidence of the condition is greater in older mares; however there is not universal agreement over the factors involved, although they include:

- Pneumovagina. This can occur in maiden mares with a small vulva which is dorsal to the pelvic floor, but most commonly it is caused by forward migration of the anus in older and/or thin mares. The dorsal commissure of the vulva is pulled forwards and the increased length of potential vulval orifice above the floor of the pelvis allows the aspiration of air and faecal material.
- It has been postulated that failure to resolve endometritis was due to an acquired immunological deficit in the uterine response. However, the results of experimental studies do not support this theory and a relationship between the occurrence of persistent endometritis and the presence of endometrial lesions in older mares has not been established.
- Impaired drainage of exudate through the cervix is currently thought to be the most likely explanation for persistent endometritis. Lesions which: cause 'pockets' in the uterus, interfere with myometrial contractility or prevent complete cervical relaxation may all be involved in the impaired drainage 'syndrome'.

(b) A yeast, probably *Candida (Monilia)* spp. This infection can be difficult to treat succesfully. The organism can often be isolated from all parts of the tubular tract, so these areas must be included in the treatment regime.

(c) A fungus, probably *Aspergillus* spp. This organism is more usually a cause of placentitis and abortion. The mare described in the question had foaled with no complications late in the previous breeding season and had not subsequently been mated.

47 (a) The cause of epistaxis is a progressive ethmoidal haematoma which can be seen pushing forward from the ethmoturbinate region into the nasal meati. The appearance of the lesions can vary from orange to grey/green to maroon. Sometimes the lesions cause obstruction of the nasal airways. Apart from endoscopy, sometimes by direct inspection into the sinus compartments, radiography is often helpful. *Figure 270A* is a lateral radiograph showing a discrete opacity rostral to the 'onion' of the ethmoid.

(b) Some claim that simple rupture of the lesions leads to regression, but the most widely accepted treatment is total resection. This is likely to involve the creation of a frontal osteoplastic flap to gain access to the area. *Figure 270B* shows the site 3 months after treatment. There is no evidence of recurrence but the ethmoturbinates remain deformed reflecting the expansive nature of the original lesion. Transendoscopic laser coagulation offers a future treatment possibility.

(c) Progressive ethmoidal haematoma is often multifocal and also shows a tendency to recur. Thus, the prognosis can never be better than cautiously optimistic.

48 (a) This animal has been affected for several months. There is considerable atrophy of the muscles in the elbow region of the right forelimb and secondary deformity of the left forelimb.
(b) The primary problem is affecting the right forelimb.
(c) Radial paralysis, brachial plexus neuropathy, fracture of the olecranon, carpal contracture.
(d) There has been secondary overloading of the left forelimb which has resulted in a varus deformity of the carpus.

49 (a) Intestinal neoplasia should be suspected. The commonest small intestinal tumour in the horse is lymphosarcoma, which may originate from the local lymphoid tissue in the bowel. The tumour most frequently takes the form of diffuse neoplastic invasion of the intestinal mucosa resulting in a state of malabsorption, but less commonly it can have a focal distribution resulting in partial bowel obstruction. Other tumours that have been identified in this site include adenocarcinomas and leiomyomas/leiomyosarcomas.
(b) The prognosis in these cases is very poor, especially in the case of lymphosarcomas and adenocarcinomas. Surgical removal of a leiomyoma/leiomyosarcoma is theoretically possible; leiomyosarcomas in domestic animals generally only show local invasion of tissues and are slow to metastasise to distant sites.

50 (a) Oedema/swelling of the forelimbs, brisket and ventral neck. The jugular vein is engorged.
(b) The most likely causes of the observed clinical signs are a cranial thoracic mass (probably lymphosarcoma), congestive cardiac failure or possibly purpura haemorrhagica. There are no indications that any of the conditions are of infectious origin and although purpura haemorrhagica has been associated with previous *Streptococcus equi* infection it is unusual that more than one horse is affected. It is therefore most unlikely that other horses will be similarly affected.
(c) Auscultation and percussion of the thorax might identify fluid accumulations, areas of dullness or cardiac defects. Radiography, ultrasonography and thoracocentesis should be employed to aid the diagnosis.
- Assessment of heart rate and character of the pulse.
- Auscultation of the heart: Are there any abnormal sounds? Do the heart sounds radiate over the normal area? Is there an audible or palpable thrill?
- Auscultation of the lungs: Are there any abnormal lung sounds? Are lung sounds audible over the normal extent of both lung fields?
- Percussion of the thorax: is there an area of dullness due to a localised mass and/or accumulation of fluid?
- Ultrasonographic examination of the heart and lungs: Is heart function normal? Can a thoracic mass or pleural fluid be identified?
- Radiographic examination: Is the heart of normal size? Are the lungs normally aerated? Is there evidence of a thoracic mass and/or fluid accumulation?
- Thoracocentesis: If there is free pleural fluid, is it an exudate, transudate, blood or lymph? Are there any abnormal cells?

51 (a) Rectal examination (*Figure 271A*) suggests the presence of an enlarged and impacted caecum. This needs to be differentiated from impactions in other viscera such as the right dorsal colon (colic ampulla) and right ventral colon, and from caecocolic intussusception.

(b) Both medical and surgical management have been advocated. The clinician's choice is guided by the rectal findings since clinical signs can be mild even in the most severe cases. If the impaction is small and easily indented, medical management (starvation, oral liquid paraffin, oral and intravenous fluids) is recommended.

(c) The caecum is much more likely to rupture with accumulation of ingesta than any other part of the large intestine. In a recent study (Campbell, 1984) the duration of clinical signs before rupture ranged from 4 to 96 h.

(d) In view of the danger of acute rupture, surgery should be considered as soon as rectal findings suggest a very large caecum or an impaction of a near-hard consistency.

Surgical intervention consists of:

- Laparotomy (*Figure 271B*) with softening and massaging of the impacted mass, or
- Typhlotomy at the caecal apex with evacuation of the impacted contents.
- Caecocolic or ileocolic anastomosis to facilitate ingesta flow pass the caecum.

52 (a) Atrial fibrillation. There are no P waves present. The isoelectric line shows coarse undulations characteristic of f waves. The R–R interval is irregular.

(b) The movement of the anterior mitral valve leaflet is abnormal. The mitral valve opens normally during rapid filling (the E point) but there is no A point. The A point is normally associated with atrial contraction. The distance between the interventricular septum and the E point of the anterior mitral valve motion is normal. This suggests that there is no enlargement of the left ventricle. (*Figure 272*, the normal situation, is shown here for comparison, with A and E points marked.)

(c) Oral administration of quinidine sulphate is the recommended treatment. A dose of 10 mg/kg is given initially to test for idiosyncratic reactions. Therapy is then continued at 20 mg/kg every 2 h until there is conversion to a normal sinus rhythm or toxic signs occur. A maximum dose of 60–80 g is given. If conversion to a normal sinus rhythm is not achieved, the process can be repeated 48 h later. Quinidine can be administered by the intravenous route as the glucuronate.

(d) The presence of any underlying cardiac disease must be determined. Horses with significant cardiac disease are less likely to convert to normal sinus rhythm than horses with no evidence of cardiac disease. Careful auscultation is important to determine any underlying valvular disease. Horses with resting heart rates in excess of 60 beats/min and other signs of congestive cardiac failure should not be treated. An accurate history is also helpful. Horses with a longstanding history of atrial fibrillation are less likely to convert to normal sinus rhythm and in those that do convert the arrhythmia is more likely to recur. Horses with no underlying cardiac disease and a recent history of atrial fibrillation are more likely to respond to treatment. Echocardiography is useful in assessing the severity of any underlying cardiac disease prior to treatment.

53 (a) This is a case of chondritis affecting the left arytenoid (to the right in *Figure 44*). The major feature is the axial displacement of the cartilage which allows the palatal pillar to be seen between the aryepiglottic fold and the pharyngeal wall. In some instances contact lesions will be visible on the medial face of the contralateral arytenoid or there may be an exuberance where sinus tracts open from the micro-abscesses within the cartilage matrix. Unilateral aryteroid chondritis represents an important clinical and endoscopic differential diagnosis for recurrent laryngeal neuropathy (hemiplegia). In both conditions the horse will produce stridor at exercise although, in addition, some horses with chondritis cough. On endoscopy the affected arytenoid will intrude into the airway in both disorders but the features mentioned above should help to differentiate

between them. However, particular vigilance is required when symptoms develop in a horse which was previously eupnoeic.
(b) Medical therapy using potentiated sulphonamides is of some value in fresh cases but will be futile once the condition is established to the stage where the cricoarytenoid articulation has ankylosed. Thereafter the only options are surgical and consist of partial or subtotal arytenoidectomy, i.e. the diseased cartilage is resected.

54 (a) When the original injury occurred this ventral rupture of the abdominal wall may have been obscured by local haemorrhage and oedema. However, when the area is auscultated, borborygmi should be louder in this region than over other areas of the abdomen. If within reach, intestine may be palpated per rectum passing through the acquired defect in the body wall. In this chronic case, direct palpation may define a fibrous ring formed by the muscular defect.
(b) Open reduction and repair of the abdominal wall defect. If the muscle damage is extensive, prosthetic mesh implantation may be used.
(c) Polypropylene, stainless steel and woven nylon are all of low reactivity, are inert in the presence of infection and produce the least incidence of postoperative discharge.
● Polypropylene is easily handled, of high tensile strength and produces the least number of adhesions when extraperitoneal placement is not possible.
● Woven nylon is cheaper, maintains good rigidity, but is prone to fraying when cut.
● Stainless steel is associated with an increased incidence of adhesions (compared to polypropylene) if directly apposed to intestinal wall.
● A compatible monofilament suture material should be used in association with each type of prosthetic material.

55 (a) Obstruction of the venous return or lymphatic drainage from the forequarters and head of the horse without affecting the caudal circulatory efficiency could result in this distribution of oedema. This could be due to a cranial thoracic or mediastinal mass. Congestive heart failure should also be excluded but is usually not associated with marked weight loss. A mass such as an abscess or tumour may be responsible for marked weight loss. Weight loss may be associated with hypoproteinaemia and secondary oedema, but the latter is usually more generalised than in this example.
(b) Intermittent pyrexic episodes lasting from 1 to 4 days are frequently encountered in cases of lymphosarcoma and internal abscessation which are the most likely differential diagnoses for the clinical signs. Pyrexia may be missed unless rectal temperature is measured repeatedly throughout the day.

56 (a) This foal is showing signs of multiple organ infections, suggesting immune deficiency. The breed (i.e. Arabian) and absolute lymphopenia are highly suggestive of combined immunodeficiency syndrome (CID). Three criteria are necessary to confirm a diagnosis of CID: absence of serum IgM; absolute lymphopenia; evidence of diffuse hypoplasia of lymphoid tissues examined post-mortem.
CID is a primary immune deficiency disease characterised by an absence of both B- and T-lymphocytes. Affected foals appear normal at birth, and remain free of clinical signs until maternal immunoglobulins (i.e. colostrum-derived immunoglobulins) wane.
(b) The foal is showing clinical signs suggestive of infections of the alimentary tract, respiratory tract and skin. Cryptosporidia are important causes of enteropathy in a number of species, including immunocompromised individuals (e.g. humans affected by AIDS). Infection with these protozoa results in stunting and fusion of small intestinal villi. Other pathogens, including bacteria and viruses, may also be involved. Respiratory

infections are common in cases of CID; infections by adenovirus, *Pneumocystis carinii* and various bacteria can be involved. The radiographic changes in this foal's lungs confirm the presence of pneumonia. This foal is also infected by *Dermatophilus congolensis*, causing skin lesions.

57 Progesterone concentrations in peripheral blood (plasma) start to rise immediately after ovulation and are usually greater than 1 ng/ml between 2 and 14 days after ovulation during a normal cycle: in cases of prolonged dioestrus these luteal progesterone values are maintained for as long as the corpus luteum persists. Modern (Elisa) tests for progesterone can be performed in any laboratory in a few hours. However, reliance on this test wastes time and money and should rarely be required by a clinician who is experienced in interpreting the anatomical (and particularly ultrasonographical) changes in the reproductive tract.

58 (a)
● Chronic granulation tissue.
● Granulomatous sarcoid.
● Fungal granuloma.
(b)
● Radical surgical excision.
● Treatment with escharotics such as concentrated lotagen or copper sulphate.
● Cryosurgery.
● While fungal granulomas do respond to surgery and sodium iodide IV, they can recur if not fully removed.
(c) Prognosis should be very guarded:
● Sarcoids in this region are refractory to treatment.
● The area is prone to injury and so continued chronic granulation is likely.
● Deeper structures – wall of foot, cartilage of the foot – are likely to be damaged.

59 (a) No (focal retinal degeneration).
(b) Areas of increased reflectivity, change in colour and pigmentary disturbance with normal retina above and between.

60 (a) These lesions, as in this instance, are usually on the axial surface of the medial malleolus and are most favourably viewed in dorsoplantar projections. They may also be seen in dorsolateral–plantaromedial oblique projections.
(b)
● Distal intermediate ridge of tibia.
● Lateral trochlear ridge of talus.
● Medial malleolus of tibia.
● Medial trochlear ridge of talus.

61 (a) Cauda equina neuritis, equine rhinopneumonitis virus (Equine Herpes Virus 1, EHV1) and sorghum poisoning may result in signs which are broadly similar. Other possibilities are very rare.
(b) Given the preceding upper respiratory tract infection, EHV1 is the most likely diagnosis. This causes an upper respiratory tract syndrome and a neurological syndrome which is attributed to an ischaemic vasculitis resulting in paresis. It is also a cause of abortion. Cauda equina syndrome is a rare idiopathic condition.

(c) The prognosis in cases of EHV1, neurological syndrome is dependent on the extent of the damage and the duration of the paralysis. Careful nursing and supportive measures may allow time for a complete recovery. The prognosis in cases of idiopathic cauda equina syndrome is generally hopeless although affected horses may be nursed by emptying the rectum and bladder over short periods.

62 (a) The pony is showing signs of weight loss associated with hypoalbuminaemia. The elevated SAP probably does not relate to liver disease, since the other liver enzymes and results of BSP clearance test are normal; raised SAP levels may occur in some cases of bowel and bone disease. In the absence of any evidence of hepatic or renal disease, the most likely cause of the hypoalbuminaemia is intestinal tract disease resulting in malabsorption and/or protein-losing enteropathy.
(b) The next logical diagnostic step would be to perform an oral glucose tolerance test to assess small intestinal absorptive capacity. If this is abnormal, then bowel wall biopsy may be necessary to confirm the nature of the disease.

63 (a) Low values of plasma albumin; high values of plasma globulin, in particular of beta globulin.
(b) Strongylosis – most probably typhlitis/colitis due to the presence of cyathostome larvae within the mucosa. A specific syndrome of seasonal (spring) diarrhoea and weight loss is seen most often in young adults and is referred to as larval cyathostomiasis. However, cyathostome larvae can also accumulate in very large numbers in older animals and may result in a chronic protein-losing enteropathy. Large or small strongyle infections often cause a serum globulin response, particularly of the gamma globulin IgG(T) which migrates in the beta globulin protein fraction during electrophoresis.
(c) Histopathological examination of large intestinal biopsy specimens will allow definitive differentiation from other protein-losing enteropathies, such as alimentary lymphosarcoma and inflammatory enteritides, which may have a very similar clinical presentation and plasma biochemical abnormalities.
(d) Larvicidal doses of anthelmintic, e.g. ivermectin at 0.2 mg/kg, oxfendazole at 10–50 mg/kg, or fenbendazole at 30 mg/kg as a single dose or at 7.5 mg/kg as five consecutive daily doses. Cyathostome larvae inhibited in development within the intestinal mucosa are not killed by anthelmintics and animals with cyathostome typhlitis/colitis should be dosed with an anthelmintic at 2- or 3-weekly intervals. Some of these cases may benefit from corticosteroid therapy, e.g. prednisolone at 1 mg/kg body weight daily (mornings) by mouth. It is thought that in addition to their anti-inflammatory effect, corticosteroids may modulate the host response to the mucosal parasites such that larvae resume development from a hypobiotic state and therefore become susceptible to the action of anthelmintics. The corticosteroid therapy should be on a reducing dose over about 3 weeks. Symptomatic treatment for diarrhoea, e.g. codeine phosphate orally at a dose rate of 1 mg/kg body weight twice daily, is also indicated.
  The prognosis in cases of parasitic typhlitis/colitis is fair to good.

64 (a) Only skin has dehisced. This will heal by secondary intention and therefore can be managed conservatively. Keep the wound clean and dress it daily to remove old crusts. Consider applying an antimicrobial skin cream, preferably without corticosteroids which may delay wound healing.

(b) Very slight. There is a good healing reaction in the muscle layer and unless abscessation occurs on the suture line, healing should proceed normally.

65 (a) Rectal examination should reveal distended loops of small intestine. The presence of finger-thick, fleshy cords entering one of the inguinal rings and tender to traction should also be noted (*Figure 273*).
(b) Diagnosis is of acute small intestinal obstruction, which has resulted from strangulation of a loop of bowel in an inguinal canal.
(c) The effusion of abnormal peritoneal fluid may have been trapped within the inguinal canal. This resulted in a normal sample on paracentesis.
(d) Immediate exploratory laparotomy is advised to reduce the hernia and remove devitalised bowel. A second incision is made directly over the inguinal ring to aid with reduction. Bilateral castration and surgical closure of the external inguinal ring should be considered.

66 (a) There is spinal cord disease between L2 and L6 with lower motor neurone (ventral grey matter) involvement on the right side resulting in neurogenic muscle atrophy.
(b) Equine protozoal myeloencephalitis (EPM) is the most likely cause and very few other diseases could mimic this syndrome. Slowly progressive verminous myelitis or an epidural lymphosarcoma could be given some consideration.
(c) The current therapy for *Sarcocystis neurona*, the putative cause of EPM, is 15 mg/kg of trimethoprim/sulphadiazine combination b.i.d., and 0.25 mg/kg of pyrimethamine s.i.d., for an initial period of 6 weeks, Most neurologists agree that such therapy can kill *S. neurona in vivo*, however the prognosis depends on the site(s), extent and severity of the neuronal loss.

67 (a) Radiography should be performed to establish the presence of any bony abnormalities. Ultrasonography is useful to establish the extent (depth) of the swelling and its relationship to the cervical vertebrae. Aspiration may be indicated for bacterial culture and sensitivity testing.
(b) Immediate pain, heat swelling and stiffness would be seen. Local clostridial infection might be a significant and potentially fatal complication.
(c) Soft tissue mineralisation and neurological deficits might arise and a permanent disability is possible.

68 (a) There is distension of the femoropatellar joint capsule, and a very upright stance on the right hindlimb associated with mild flexural deformity of the metatarsophalangeal (fetlock) joint.
(b) Both clinical signs relate to conditions associated with rapid growth in animals on a high plane of nutrition.
(c) Osteochondrosis dissecans of the lateral trochlear ridge of the distal femur, and flexural deformity of the fetlock joint associated with relative shortening of the superficial flexor tendon.
(d) The animal's diet should be investigated with particular reference to energy and protein concentrations and mineral balance. Its nutritional plane should be reduced. The owner should be alerted to the problem so that, ideally, it can be avoided in other young stock and, if not avoided, recognised at the earliest stage possible. Although osteochondrosis is not heritable, predisposing factors may be, so avoid breeding from the same mare–stallion combination.

69 (a) *Taylorella equigenitalis* and *Klebsiella pneumoniae* (certain capsule types only) are bacteria known to infect the uteri of young, genitally healthy mares without there being any apparent predisposing factors. Endometritis usually persists for one or more cycles in such mares if the condition is not treated, but eventually resolution will occur. However, the mare then may become a 'carrier'; the organism can remain in the clitoral area, as a saprophyte. Various strains of *Pseudomonas aeruginosa* have also been incriminated in this role although there is no general agreement that the organism has a predilection for the mare's uterus. However, in view of the fact that is it usually resistant to routinely used antibiotics, isolation of the organism from anywhere in the reproductive tract should warrant special consideration.

Coital exanthema is caused by Equine Herpes Virus 3 (EHV3) and is transmitted during mating. EHV1 (viral abortion) is not known to be transmitted in this manner. Equine viral arteritis does not occur in Great Britain and does not cause venereal disease although it is present in the ejaculate of affected stallions.

(b) Stallions show no clinical signs due to venereal bacteria and are purely 'carriers' of the organisms. Klebsiella has been isolated from the urinary tract in a stallion.

Mares usually have a uterine discharge which is seen at the vulva, especially during early oestrus. The volume varies between copious pus seen dripping from the vulva, to small amounts of dried exudate on the underside of the tail. The discharge is not characteristic of venereal disease. After resolution of the uterine infection organisms may remain 'dormant' in the vestibular area, particularly in the clitoral fossa and sinuses. Coital exanthema causes vesicles on the vulva, vestibule and penis; these rupture to form ulcers which usually heal spontaneously. Presumably, as with other herpes viruses, latency and recrudescence occur.

(c) Swab samples are taken before the breeding season. Samples should be obtained from the stallion's urethra, urethral fossa and sheath and placed immediately into Stuart's or Amie's transport medium. Mares are swabbed from the clitoral sinus and fossa. Animals which harbour venereal pathogens are not mated until treatment has eliminated the organisms.

The regimes adopted by different countries and breed societies vary, but should be designed to prevent the spread of venereal disease. *Figure 274A* shows the clitoris and part of the surrounding fossa, within the vulval lips. The clitoral sinus opens onto the dorsal surface of the clitoris in the midline; smegma may be forced out of it by squeezing the clitoris (*Figure 274B*).

70 (a) Nodules containing larvae of *Strongylus edentatus*. In the case illustrated the larvae have been killed *in situ* following administration of an anthelmintic. As a result a fibrous reaction has developed around each larva such that the lesions are evident as discrete nodules. In untreated animals there is usually relatively little host reaction to *S. edentatus* larvae in this subperitoneal site with generally only slight, localised haemorrhage, oedema and peritoneal thickening.

(b) The *S. edentatus* larval nodules per se are not likely to be the cause of clinical signs of recurrent colic and chronic weight loss. The life-cycle of *S. edentatus* is migratory: intestine – portal system – liver – hepatorenal ligament – parietal peritoneum – intestine. At all of these sites it is frequently possible to find pathological changes of haemorrhage and inflammatory cellular infiltrates of recent migration or chronic fibrosis in later stages. However, even when such changes are marked, e.g. in the liver, they have not been associated with clinical signs in either naturally acquired or experimental infections. The presence of lesions of *S. edentatus* infection is evidence that this animal has probably ingested other strongyle larvae, and it is likely that the horse will have acquired a mixed strongyle burden. *Strongylus vulgaris* – and to a lesser extent *Cyathostomum* spp. – are well recognised as causes of colic and weight loss, and they are more likely to be the causes of the clinical signs of this case.

71 (a) Occult sarcoid, neurofibroma or other tumour.
(b) Take full skin thickness biopsy for histopathological examination, either punch biopsy or wedge biopsy.
(c) The procedure may cause rapid proliferation into a granulomatous-type sarcoid.
(d) Cryosurgery can be considered onto nodules only, or BCG injected intralesionally. Local irradiation with β-irradiation may be successful.

72 (a) The stylet has pierced the wall of the catheter. This can occur if the stylet is withdrawn and then readvanced whilst the catheter is left in place either in the vein or in the subcutaneous tissues.
(b) Perivascular injection of an irritant substance could have occurred. Alternatively, the end of the catheter could have been sheared off, resulting in an embolism which may have caused problems, e.g. coronary arterial occlusion, pulmonary embolism, depending on the anatomical site at which it lodged.

73 Difficulty in palpating the whole reproductive tract can be contributed to by:
● Inexperience of the clinician.
● Inadequate restraint of the mare.
● Excessive straining of the mare.
However, even under conditions that are close to ideal, palpation of an ovary may be difficult. This is usually because the ovary which is suspended in the cranial border of the broad ligament is lying lateral to this ligament, which makes it impossible to palpate any detail of the ovary. Returning the ovary to a position medial to the broad ligament can be difficult. One method is to pass a finger round the utero-ovarian ligament, ventral to the ovary, and gently press upwards. This usually causes the ovary to rotate medially where it then becomes clearly palpable. Most clinicians find the left ovary the more difficult to palpate if they use their left hand, and vice versa.

74 (a) An umbilical hernia may be classified by its:
● Aetiology – congenital, inherited or acquired.
● Behaviour – reducible, irreducible.
● Contents – fat, omentum, intestines.
● Size.
● Location – umbilical.
(b)
● The animal's age and the size of the hernial ring – the majority of small to medium size hernias will close spontaneously as the foal gets older, therefore surgical interference should be delayed until 6–12 months of age. Larger defects are, however, more easily closed as early as possible.
● Presence of infection – is the hernia associated with omphalophlebitis? This may be confirmed either by needle aspiration or ultrasound.
● Are the hernial sac contents reducible?
(c)
● Open reduction – under general anaesthesia an elliptical piece of skin is dissected free from the hernial sac without penetrating the peritoneum. The peritoneal sac is freed

from its attachments to the defect in the abdominal wall and returned to the abdomen. Heavy synthetic absorbable suture material may be used to close the abdominal wall defect using either a Mayo ('vest over pants') or single interrupted patterns. The skin is closed routinely.

Large defects may require prosthetic mesh implantation. For maximum mechanical advantage, the mesh should be placed in an extraperitoneal position beneath the rectus sheath. A fascial overlay technique with the mesh in an intraperitoneal position has been used to reduce postoperative seroma formation.

- Closed reduction – the hernial contents are reduced and clamps placed across the pendulous skin, to treat cosmetically the hernia. This traditional technique has the potential to lead to complications such as intestinal entrapment.

(d) Unless an acquired aetiology can be determined, umbilical hernias are considered an inheritable defect and the animal should be removed from any breeding programme.

75 Starting at about 100 days of gestation the fetal gonads, irrespective of whether they are potentially testes or ovaries, start to produce increasing quantities of oestrogens. Concentrations in blood and urine reach a maximum at about 150 d and these values are maintained until around 300 d; thereafter concentrations slowly decrease. The main oestrogens produced are oestrone, equilin and equilenin, the latter two being peculiar to equine pregnancy.

The function of these hormones in pregnancy is unclear, although they do not induce the mare to show signs of oestrus, even though blood concentrations are many times greater than when the mare is in oestrus during normal cycles. The cervix of the pregnant mare softens in the latter half of pregnancy, which may be related to oestrogen production, but relaxation and opening do not occur.

For many years the 'urine test' has been used to diagnose pregnancy. The Cuboni and Lunaas tests involve a colour reaction when large quantities of oestrogen are present in the urine. More recently radioimmunoassays have been used to measure oestrone sulphate in plasma. The oestrone is conjugated in the fetal liver so that a large concentration of oestrone sulphate indicates fetal viability.

76 (a) Lateromedial, dorsopalmar, dorsoproximal–palmarodistal oblique and dorsolateral–palmaromedial oblique views.
(b) The view in *Figure 62A* is not a true lateromedial projection; no significant radiographic abnormality can be detected. No significant abnormalities can be detected in *Figures 62B* and C.
(c) Palmaroproximal–palmarodistal oblique view.
(d) There is an incomplete non-displaced fracture through the medial palmar process of the distal phalanx.

Treatment: box rest; apply a bar shoe and reassess clinically and radiographically after 6 weeks.

Prognosis: fair; a bony union cannot be guaranteed.

77 (a) Only the white and thinly haired areas are affected, which is suggestive of photosensitisation. Causes of photosensitisation include congenital porphyria, ingestion of plants containing photodynamic agents (e.g. St John's wort) and hepatic disease. Since the horse shows chronic weight loss, hepatic disease is the most likely diagnosis.
(b) Photosensitisation in hepatic failure is caused by failure of excretion of phylloerythrin, a metabolite of chorophyll. Phylloerythrin accumulates in the skin where it acts as a photodynamic agent.

78 (a) The clinical findings are suggestive of a pleural effusion. There are numerous potential causes of pleural effusions, and the types of fluid fall into the general categories of transudate, exudate, haemorrhage and chyle. Most effusions in the horse are transudative, or exudative in nature. Exudative effusions are commonly associated with pleuritis secondary to pneumonia or lung abscesses. Transudative effusions are most often associated with neoplasia.

(b) Radiography and diagnostic ultrasound may both be used to confirm the presence of an effusion, and they may also provide some information concerning the underlying disease process. The nature of the pleural fluid should be assessed by analysis of a sample obtained by thoracocentesis. Cell counts, cytology, and estimations of protein and glucose concentrations are useful in determining the precise nature of the fluid. Bacteriological culture (aerobic and anaerobic) should be performed in cases of septic exudates.

79 The palatal arch is dorsally displaced so that the epiglottis is not visible. This was the position throughout a prolonged endoscopic inspection of the pharynx and larynx and in spite of multiple deglutition sequences. The cause of the persistent DDSP can be attributed to two intrapalatal cysts both lying approximately 1 cm from the rostral margin of the arcus palatopharyngeus. The larger is on the horse's left (right in *Figure 275*). Intrapalatal cysts are not common and are thought to arise from salivary tissue in the palatal mucosa. Surgical resection of the cysts is not easy because of poor access both from the mouth or via a laryngotomy. In addition, chronic fistulation through the palate is a likely sequel, especially when the cysts are as large as those illustrated.

80 (a) There is excessive exuberant granulation tissue, a common complication found at this site. The aim is to reduce this granulation tissue. It may be possible to debulk this partially by sharp dissection. Granulation tissue does not have a nerve supply but profuse haemorrhage may occur! The owner can apply cortisone antibiotic emollient creams daily to reduce the granulation tissue until the wound heals.

(b) Many take up to 12–18 months. Constant motion at the wound site is a problem.

(c) There will be an area of hard fibrous tissue on the dorsal aspect of the hock, which, with vigorous exercises, may be subject to further injury. Unless there is any underlying bony abnormality, there is generally no gait abnormality due to the fibrous tissue per se.

81 Refer to *Figure 276*.

(a) Traction or avulsion of the insertion of the suspensory ligament.

(b) Ultrasonographic evaluation of the suspensory ligament: serious suspensory ligament pathology will warrant a much more guarded prognosis.

(c) Removal is generally indicated for apical fractures which are up to one-third of the proximodistal distance of the bone.

82 (a) Larval cyathostomiasis. There is congestion and oedema of the colonic mucosa and many, small dark lesions are evident which represent mucosal cyathostome larvae.

(b) It is often possible to identify the presence of the causative parasites by gross inspection of faeces, e.g. on a rectal sleeve after palpation of abdominal organs. The worms vary in size from about 2–7 mm and are either red or white in colour.

At necropsy, transillumination of the gut wall will allow confirmation of the presence of mucosal cyathostomes. Ideally this procedure should be performed on sections of separated mucosa with a strong white light and magnification, but even without such facilities it is possible to identify multiple, minute larvae within the tissue by use of any available light source, e.g. a strong torch.

Histopathological examination of fixed biopsy specimens collected either at exploratory laparotomy or post-mortem examination should give definitive confirmation of the diagnosis.

(c) Inhibition of development of cyathostome larvae within the large intestinal mucosa is pivotal to the pathogenesis of the clinical syndrome of larval cyathostomiasis. The details of the biological mechanisms which result in inhibited development of these parasites are not known, but it would appear that it is a manifestation of partial host immunity to cyathostome infection.

The onset of clinical signs occurs when there is synchronous, mass emergence of large numbers of mucosal larvae. The principal effect of the pathological events is a protein-losing enteropathy such that severely affected animals usually exhibit marked, rapid weight loss and often develop peripheral oedema.

83 (a) The filly has an intact hymen. She has probably become reproductively active recently and uterine secretions are accumulating cranial to the hymen so that at times when intrapelvic pressure is increased, the membrane bulges between the vulval lips.

Examination reveals that the hand cannot be passed further into the tract than the level of the urethra. In most cases, pressure in the centre of the obstruction with a forefinger causes rupture of the hymen and forward progression of the hand dilates the canal. No pain is evident and haemorrhage, if any, is minimal. Sometimes the hymen is so tough that it must be grasped with tissue forceps, retracted and incised with a scalpel blade or hypodermic needle; thereafter a finger may be inserted as previously described.

(b) This occurs usually in mares that are foaling for the first time. Probably the foal's toe catches on a dorsal remnant of hymen at the vestibulovaginal junction and because of continued straining the foot is forced through the dorsal vaginal wall and into the rectum. Occasionally, repositioning of the foal due to relaxation and possibly rolling by the mare, caused the limb to retract and thereafter follow the normal route of expulsion. The lesion thus formed heals and leaves the mare with a rectovaginal fistula. If, however, penetration of the rectum is followed by continued straining of the mare, a rectovestibular tear occurs up to and through the perineum.

Initial treatment is tetanus antitoxin if the mare has not been vaccinated; antibiotic treatment may be given but is not usually necessary. The lesion should then be left to granulate. Trying to reappose the damaged tissues is not successful due to post-traumatic necrosis, oedema and sepsis. The mare cannot be covered during this breeding season. It is usually convenient to delay surgery until the foal has been weaned. Reconstruction of the area is difficult and may require several attempts. Surgery may be carried out under epidural anaesthesia.

84 Colour codes and general usage of venous blood evacuated container systems:

Stopper colour	Tube contents	General usage
Violet	EDTA	Haematology
Blue	Sodium citrate (3.8%)	Fibrinogen (Clauss method), and coagulation studies

Black	Sodium citrate (3.1%)	Erythrocyte sedimentation rate (ESR) (of limited value in the horse)
Grey	Sodium fluoride–potassium oxalate	Glucose
Red	Plain (no anticoagulant)	Serum biochemistry
Green	Lithium heparin	Plasma endocrinology, fibrinogen (heat precipitation method)

85 (a) Bacterial endocarditis.
(b) There is no one feature that is pathognomonic of bacterial endocarditis. Diagnosis is based on the presence of some of the following signs. There is usually a heart murmur which may be recent in onset. Damage to the valve usually results in regurgitant murmurs, although the presence of a large vegetation on a semilunar valve may result in a systolic ejection murmur. Dysrhythmias may be present due to myocarditis. Bacteraemia may result in persistent or recurrent fever; anorexia, depression and polyarthritis may develop. Haematology may show anaemia and leucocytosis. Two or more positive blood cultures are strongly suggestive of bacterial endocarditis.
(c) Antibiotic treatment should be given based on sensitivity results from positive blood cultures if available. Ideally intravenous therapy should be given. Long-term therapy is necessary initially for 1 month and then re-culture is advised. Bacteriocidal drugs are preferable.
(d) The outcome is dependent on the degree of cardiac damage at the onset of treatment and the success of antibacterial therapy. Prompt treatment of acute bacterial endocarditis may result in mild cardiac dysfunction. However, organisation of vegetations and the deposition of fibrin makes the elimination of bacteria difficult. This results in chronic damage and deformation of valve structures. Thromboembolism and immune complexes may result in damage to other organ systems.

86 The horse has sustained an avulsion fracture of the nuchal crest of the occipital bone. Note also the mineralisation caudal to the nuchal crest (not itself of clinical significance). Conservative management is likely to be successful as a fibrous union will form within a few weeks and the horse will recover a normal range of neck mobility. During the early stages of recovery all food should be provided at ground level and water offered from a shallow vessel if there is no natural water source. The horse can be assisted to maintain its head in a raised position with pillar chains once the acute reaction has settled down.

87 (a) On one side of the foot the heel of the shoe is resting on the seat of corn. If the animal is not already lame, this may cause lameness as a result of bruising in this region.
(b) The owner should have the animal adequately shod with sufficient heel cover. The heels of this shoe look relatively short in comparison to the shape of the foot, but this is partly because to the fact that the animal has not been shod for some time. Therefore, the owner should help the farrier by having the animal shod at more appropriate intervals, perhaps every 4 weeks depending upon the rate of hoof growth.

88 (a) No (peripapillary retinal degeneration).
(b) Finger-like pale projections with pigmentary disturbance on both sides of the optic disc.

89 (a) Equine sarcoid due to a virus which is not yet categorised; may be related to bovine papilloma virus.
(b) Yes. Flies and blood from injured lesion are capable of spreading similar disease to other horses.
(c) Many of this type of sarcoid remain quiescent if untouched. Surgical excision is not the best treatment due to the spread of 'virus' during surgery into normal tissue.
(d) There would be success in approximately 50% of cases up to 2 years after surgery.

90 The characteristic site for discharge from a temporal teratoma is at the base of the pinna. The term temporal teratoma is preferred to dentigerous cyst because occasional dermoid teratomas occur without dental tissue being present. Radiographs are helpful, first to discover whether the teratoma contains dental tissue and second to determine the site and size of the lesion. The lesion should be removed surgically. The surgical removal of a temporal teratoma depends upon following the sinus tract to its base, followed by removal of the dermoid or dental material. Some dental lesions are large and firmly attached to the petrous temporal bone.

91 (a) The clinical signs and history, and the clinical pathological findings suggest a diagnosis of peritonitis. There is leucocytosis with neutrophilia, and hyperfibrinogenaemia indicative of a severe inflammatory reaction. The total nucleated cell and neutrophil counts in the peritoneal fluid are grossly elevated indicating peritonitis. Examination of Gram-stained smears of peritoneal fluid may reveal bacteria in such cases.
(b) Peritonitis may have many different underlying causes, but the commonest causes of spontaneous peritonitis (i.e. unrelated to surgical interference of the abdomen) in adult horses relate to bowel wall damage (e.g. ulceration/infarction/foreign body/perforation, etc.).
(c) Treatment with broad-spectrum, bactericidal antiobiotics is indicated; use of metronidazole may be considered. Culture of peritoneal fluid and antibiotic sensitivity testing should be attempted, although this often fails to produce any isolates. Symptomatic therapy with non-steroidal anti-inflammatory drugs (e.g. flunixin meglumine), analgesics, and fluid and electrolytes may be required. Long-term therapy (many weeks) is often necessary. The progress of the case can be usefully monitored by sequential analysis of blood samples (haematology and fibrinogen) and peritoneal fluid (cell count).
   Exploratory laparotomy may be indicated in horses showing signs of severe pain, or cases that fail to respond to medical treatment.

92 This is probably a form of lymphoid neoplasia, possibly a true lymphocytic leukaemia. The haematological abnormalities are the result of myelophthisis, i.e. invasion and replacement of the normal marrow elements by neoplastic cells. Tumour cell proliferation proceeds at the expense of normal haematopoiesis, resulting in a decrease in many of the marrow-derived cells in the circulation. This explains the anaemia, neutropenia and thrombocytopenia. The latter is the likely cause of the clinical features of mucosal haemorrhages and epistaxis. Cytological examination of blood smears may reveal abnormal forms of lymphoid cells (such as lymphoblasts, large lymphocytes, etc.). Confirmation of the diagnosis should be possible by examination of the bone marrow (obtained by biopsy/aspiration).

93 (a) There are longitudinal ulcers of the oesophageal mucosa, probably the result of reflux from the stomach into the oesophagus.

(b) Grass sickness (equine dysautonomia). A generalised alimentary tract paralysis is generally found. In more acute cases the most significant lesions are associated with the small intestine and stomach, while in chronic cases there is more effect upon the large colon. While most cases are associated with grazing horses in summer the disease has (rarely) been found under other conditions.

(c) A definitive diagnosis can usually be made by identifying the characteristic chromatolysis within the ganglia of the autonomic nervous system. Usually the cranial sympathetic ganglia are obtained but there is no necessity to be so restricted.

(d) While an aetiological agent has not yet been identified the disease may occur in groups of grazing horses in limited areas of the world. The owner should be aware of this possibility, though what measures the owner could take to prevent the disease are not known!

94 (a) It is not uncommon for mares as young as 5 years old to be affected, but most are 7–12 years old when the tumour is diagnosed.

(b) Granulosa cell tumours are said to cause either persistent oestrus, persistent anoestrus or masculinisation (virilism). The last syndrome is the most common and is characterised by stallion-like behaviour, including 'teasing' mares and mounting; testosterone concentrations in plasma are elevated. This variety of clinical signs suggests that not all tumours diagnosed as granulosa cell tumours are endocrinologically similar, and they may differ histologically as well. The terms 'gynandroblastoma' and 'sex cord stromal cell tumour' have been suggested to try to avoid the problems involved in classifying these tumours accurately.

(c)
- Abnormal clinical behaviour.
- Palpable findings (per rectum) are that the affected ovary is usually in excess of 10 cm diameter, is roughly spherical and has a smooth surface; however, granulosa cell tumours are usually larger than this and may reach 25 cm diameter (*Figure 277A*) with the same superficial characteristics as the small tumours. Whether or not the larger tumours are advanced stages of the smaller ones is not known. In all cases the whole ovary is neoplastic. An additional diagnostic feature is that the non-affected ovary is small, hard and completely inactive.
- Ultrasonographically small tumours may be solid (*Figure 277B*) or contain many cavities which may be circular or wedge-shaped and are usually of a similar size (0.5–1.5 cm) (*Figure 277C*). Scanning confirms the overall spherical or slightly oblong shape of the ovary. Larger tumours contain larger cavities which may contain echodense lines and trabeculae, presumably caused by haemorrhage into the cavities. The largest tumours normally contain a single cavity. In places the wall of the tumour may be very thin. Subsequent gross examination of these ovaries confirms the ultrasonographic findings. Examination of the other ovary reveals almost no follicular activity.

Two conditions, of unknown aetiology and significance, may mimic granulosa cell tumours, but are rare:
- A large (>12 cm diameter) ovary containing many static follicles, i.e. there is very little morphological change over many months; it is also possible that ovulations may occur from the ovary if mature follicles are close to the ovulation fossa. The opposite ovary is also active and cycling activity is normal.

- Persistent 'haematoma'. A smooth-surfaced ovary may continue to present the same palpable and ultrasonographic features for many months. On removal the ovary is found to contain blood which is only partially clotted (*Figure 277D*). The opposite ovary is active and the mare cycles normally.

Ovaries affected in either of these ways are usually removed because they are thought to be tumours, or because it is considered that the enlarged organ might interfere with parturition should the mare conceive.

(d) Ovariectomy. Small tumours can be removed via the flank but large ones should be approached via the midline. Special problems encountered are:
- Long recumbency causing muscle damage.
- Difficulty in exteriorising the ovary for effective haemostasis.
- Postoperative haemorrhage.
- Postoperative pain.

(e) If surgery-related complications are not lethal or debilitating, the unaffected ovary can be expected to resume cyclic activity and the mare can maintain a normal pregnancy. The time of resumption of cycles appears to depend on the length of time for which the non-affected ovary has been inactive, and the season of the year – a delay in excess of 1 year is not uncommon. Once cyclic activity resumes, it occurs at the same frequency (roughly once every 3 weeks) as in mares with two ovaries.

95 (a) The blood biochemical and haematological abnormalities in this case are: azotaemia, hyperkalaemia, hypernatraemia, hypocalcaemia, hypophosphataemia and neutropenia. The values for serum total protein and albumin are right at the minimum reference values.

The horse has acute renal failure, presumably as a consequence of ischaemic renal damage following haemodynamic changes associated with the colitis. However, toxic insult affecting both kidneys and gastrointestinal tract could result in these findings.

Hyperkalaemia does not commonly occur in equine acute renal failure but it is a potentially life-threatening state due to its effects on cardiac function.

(b) Urinalysis – specific gravity, casts, cells, urea and creatinine. The ratios of either urea or creatinine in urine : plasma may be helpful in differentiating pre-renal and primary renal causes of azotaemia in less severe cases.

Measurement of either sulphanilate clearance or fractional electrolyte clearance values would be of negligible value in a case with severe excretory dysfunction, as in this mare.

Renal ultrasonography may enable identification of structural abnormalities in addition to imaging calculi, neoplasia, pyelonephritis, etc., which could also give rise to renal failure.

Electrocardiographic (ECG) examination should be performed to assess the effects of hyperkalaemia on cardiac electrical conduction.

(c) In this case, extensive medical therapy is required and should be directed at the probable underlying cause, i.e. colitis, and all potentially nephrotoxic medication should be discontinued.

Intravenous fluid therapy is required for correction of electrolyte imbalances and restoration of plasma volume deficit. Frequent monitoring of plasma electrolyte levels (potassium, sodium and chloride), total protein levels and packed cell volume would be essential.

Most horses with acute tubular necrosis will have improved urinary output by restoring fluid deficit alone. However, if oliguria persists then diuresis by use of either frusemide or a 20% solution of mannitol intravenously may be necessary.

Administration of dopamine would improve renal blood flow and glomerular filtration rate and, although extreme, haemo- or peritoneal dialysis would be possible.

If sedation or analgesia are required in the management of the colitis then the use of agents such as xylazine or detomidine is indicated since they also promote urine output.

Restoration of renal function and output would probably result in correction of any renal metabolic acidosis such that intravenous administration of bicarbonate would probably be unnecessary and it should not be given unless facilities for blood gas analysis are available.

Hyperkalaemia is potentially life threatening and therefore therapy aimed at lowering extracellular potassium (K^+) levels should be undertaken. The general therapy for this animal should lower plasma K^+ levels in that expansion of extracellular fluid volume by fluid therapy will dilute plasma K^+ levels and also increase urinary K^+ excretion by improved renal perfusion. Reversal of metabolic acidosis will promote cellular K^+ uptake which can be further enhanced by administration of intravenous glucose together with regular insulin.

Administration of intravenous calcium borogluconate solution has a cardioprotectant effect by normalisation of differences between resting membrane and threshold potentials. ECG examinations should be performed regularly to monitor the effectiveness of this therapy.

(d) If urinary output can be restored and the underlying cause of acute renal failure is successfully treated, then the prognosis is fair to good. Although this mare made a complete recovery many similarly affected cases could progress into compensated chronic renal failure.

96 (a) The skin and possibly the tendon sheath and/or the superficial digital flexor tendon. The tendon and tendon sheath may be assessed by ultrasonographic examination using a 7.5 MHz transducer.

(b) Because there is differential movement of the tendon, tendon sheath and skin.

(c) Debride the granulation tissue without exposing the superficial digital flexor if possible, to minimise the risk of adhesions subsequently developing. Apply a half-limb cast to immobilise the distal limb. Provided that there are no complications the cast may be left for 4 weeks (or up to 6 weeks in more severe lacerations). Provide systemic antimicrobial therapy for 5–7 days if there is evidence of infection. (Culture the discharge and perform antimicrobial sensitivity testing at the time of debridement; alter the antimicrobial regimen initiated at the time of surgery if indicated.)

97 (a)
- Cervix – about 1 cm wide and 7 cm long and lies in the mid-pelvic area; it feels very firm, i.e is constricted tightly due to the action of progesterone.
- Uterus – body and horns are tubular and rubbery (tonic) due to contraction of the myometrium. There is a 2.5–3.0 cm swelling at the base of one (single or unilateral twin pregnancies) or both (bilateral twin pregnancy) horns. The swelling is less distinct than the rest of the tonic uterus because the surrounding uterine wall is thin; the swelling is most pronounced ventrolaterally and can therefore only be palpated by lifting the uterus gently with the tips of the fingers.
- Ovaries – usually feel active, with several follicles up to preovulatory size; the corpus luteum of pregnancy cannot be palpated.

(b)
- Cervix – as for 21 days.
- Uterus – tone is as for 21 days or more marked (intense); the pregnancy swelling is about 4.0 cm in diameter and is tense because it is fluid-filled (cf. the 'tone' of the rest of the tract).
- Ovaries – as for 21 days but usually contain more palpable follicles.

(c)
- Cervix – as for 21 days.
- Uterus – as for 32 days but the pregnancy swelling is about 8 cm in diameter and occupies the basal half of the pregnant horn. This is the latest stage at which bilateral twins can be detected by palpation.
- Ovaries – due to the synergistic effects of equine chorionic gonadotrophin and pituitary follicle stimulating hormone on the ovaries, there is marked follicular development with the formation of secondary luteal tissue. The ovaries are therefore enlarged and active.

(d)
- Cervix – as for 21 days.
- Uterus – after 60 days the chorioallantoic membrane expands rapidly to occupy the whole of the uterus by 80–85 days; this results in the uterus becoming more or less uniform distended with allantoic fluid. Per rectum, the body of the uterus is most obvious and is usually about 12 cm wide and tense due to its fluid content.
- Ovaries – usually as for 60 days but may be smaller and displaced more cranially; they remain dorsal to the uterus.

(e)
- Cervix – as for 21 days.
- Uterus – only the body is palpable; depending on the position of the uterus and other viscera it may feel like a fluid-filled viscus in which the fetus can be ballotted by tapping the dorsal surface, or it may feel relatively non-fluid filled so that the fetus is easily palpated. Parts of the fetus, e.g. head, may be identified.
- Ovaries – these are usually small and inactive at this stage and are pulled cranially and medially so that they are difficult to palpate.

(f)
- Cervix – usually a lot softer than in earlier stages of pregnancy due to the influence of the placental oestrogen which is produced at this time.
- Uterus – the fetus is easily palpated in the body of the uterus; head or forelimbs may be identified. There is very little sensation of the fluid in the uterus.
- The ovaries are quiescent and not usually palpable at this stage.

98 Simple in-and-out wiring with 24 SWG monofilament steel wire is very effective for the fixation of incisor quadrant fractures of the mandible and maxilla. The canine and the contralateral central incisor teeth provide stabilising points (*Figure 278*). Normal occlusion is checked after removal of the endotracheal tube. Absorbable sutures may be used to repair the mucosal wounds. Care should be taken to prevent laceration of the gingival or labial mucosa by the sharp ends of the wire. This can be achieved either by tucking the ends between teeth or by covering with a blob of dental wax. In mares or geldings without canine teeth a lateral stabilising point can be created by drilling a narrow tunnel through the mandible at the corresponding point. The fracture should be stabilised within 6 weeks and the wire should be removed.

99 Refer to *Figure 279.*
(a) Flexion of the carpus assists in reduction. The treatment is reduction and fixation by internal fixation. The latter is optimally achieved by the use of an AO/ASIF cortical bone screw(s) inserted in a lag technique under arthroscopic visualisation. 3.5 mm or 4.5 mm diameter screws may be employed.
(b) The radial (medial) facet of the third carpal bone.
(c) There is comminution at the fracture margin of the parent bone and dorsopalmar wear lines in the articular cartilage palmar to the fracture.

100 (a) Although exercise results in an increased food intake, the energy requirements on days of hard exercise cannot be met by the energy intake in the feed (as feed intake is limited to between 2% and 3% body weight on a dry matter basis). During hard work it is beneficial to increase the energy density of the diet, and perhaps to increase the frequency of meals. Fat has been shown to be quite well tolerated by the horse (up to 10–15% of the diet) but feed intake tends to decrease with increasing concentration. Feeding fat might prime enzymes for the metabolism of fatty acids, the main energy source during endurance riding, and therefore result in blood glucose sparing which could enhance performance.
   Fatty acids are also important for skin and coat condition. Fats have an added advantage, when substituted for carbohydrates in horses fed high amounts of feed, as there may be a reduction of the thermal load as they increase efficiency of energy utilisation without increasing heat production.
(b) Until the limitations for fuel (pyruvate and free fatty acids) transportation into mitochondria have been determined and clarified, the relative importance of fatty acids in energy production at various work intensities and durations will not be understood. At present it is believed that fatty acids are of limited importance in energy production in the sprinting animal. However, there is some limited work which suggests that increasing the oil levels in the diets of horses in hard work may help with energy utilisation and availability during training for a sprint race. The ideal proportions of fat and carbohydrate in the diet for exercise at various intensities and durations are as yet unknown.
(c) Excess can be detrimental, not only because of a decrease in feed palatability and the possibility of dietary disturbances, but also because too much fat flowing into the large intestine will tend to decrease fibre digestibility and fat utilisation. Long-chain fatty acids have limited absorption from the large intestine.
(d) Qualitative information on the relative importance of the different fatty acids and therefore the various oils is not available for the horse. Currently, oils such as soya or corn oil have been recommended to be added to the diet (up to 200–225 ml per day for a racehorse). Any oil should, however, be introduced gradually to the diet.
   The NRC 1989 suggests that dietary dry matter should include at least 0.5% linoleic acid.

101 Inhalation tracheitis, bronchitis and pneumonia are common consequences of acute oesophageal obstruction. Pools of inhaled saliva coloured by ingesta lying within the trachea at the thoracic inlet are seen in this case. If radiographs were obtained they would show areas of consolidation in the dependent lung fields. The inhalation of contaminated material does not often lead to a fatal gangrenous pneumonia. In fact, provided that a vigorous course of broad-spectrum antibiotic is administered, most patients recover in a relatively short time. This is perhaps a testament to the efficiency of the mucociliary clearance mechanism in the horse.
   In practice, acute oesophageal choke is generally managed successfully using

spasmolytic agents, and aids such as endoscopy and thoracic radiography would be regarded as unnecessary. However, the case illustrated does emphasise the need for aggressive medication in the recovery period.

102 (a) The clinical features are typical of *Streptococcus equi* infection (strangles). This could be confirmed by bacteriological culture of purulent discharge (preferably obtained from a lymph node abscess).
(b) The treatment of strangles is controversial. In the majority of cases a spontaneous recovery occurs, and antibiotic therapy is not necessary. It is believed by some that the treatment of cases with antibiotics before the maturation of abscesses can slow the speed of recovery and increase the risk of widespread lymphatic spread of infection in the body ('bastard strangles'); there is, however, little published evidence to support this view. Penicillin is the antibiotic of choice if treatment is necessary (e.g. in severe cases, and in cases with complications such as guttural pouch empyema, aspiration pneumonia, pleuritis, abdominal abscessation, etc.). Procaine penicillin G (22 000 iu/kg twice a day) may be used until 5–10 days after the disappearance of clinical signs. A higher dose may be required in cases of 'bastard strangles'. Feeding by nasogastric tube may be needed if dysphagia is severe. Anti-inflammatory drugs (e.g. phenylbutazone, flunixin meglumine) can improve the general demeanour of severe cases. In horses with dyspnoea due to pharyngeal/laryngeal compression by abscesses, a temporary tracheostomy may be required. Lancing and draining of abscesses, once mature, are helpful.
(c) Quarantine of affected horses and strict hygiene measures should be implemented to limit the spread of infection to other susceptible animals. Twice-daily monitoring of rectal temperatures and prompt therapy with penicillin of all horses with pyrexia may prevent the development of the disease at an early stage. Alternatively, a 'blanket' prophylactic treatment of all other susceptible horses may be undertaken.

103 (a) Equine coital exanthema, caused by equine herpes virus 3.
(b) Yes, by service and possibly by careless hygiene from handlers.
(c) There may be a slight reduction due to lower resistance to bacterial infection during the viral infection.

104 (a) Arterial blood pressure monitoring and ECG.
(b) Arterial blood pressure monitoring gives more information than the ECG, which just illustrates electrical activity in the heart. Blood pressure indicates whether there is an effective cardiac output, by which tissue perfusion is maintained. Depth of anaesthesia or sympathetic tone may also be implied from sequential readings. Maintenance of effective tissue perfusion is thought to reduce the incidence of postanaesthetic myopathy.

105 (a) Fistulous withers, an infection of the bursa overlying the thoracic dorsal spinous processes in this area. This condition may be associated with prior trauma.
(b) *Brucella* spp. organisms have occasionally been associated with this disorder.
(c) Radiography to determine the presence or absence of concurrent osteomyelitis. Ultrasonography to determine the extent of the abscess.
(d) Radical surgery is usually necessary. Local infections which do not involve the bursa may be amenable to local and systemic antibiotics. Both aerobic and anaerobic bacterial culture should be performed prior to initiating antimicrobial therapy. The major problem is associated with the difficulty of providing adequate drainage of the infected site.

106 (a) There is distension of the tendon sheath of the extensor carpi radialis.
(b) A good history to establish whether there has been penetration of this structure and possible infection. A clinical examination to establish what level of lameness, if any, is present, synovial fluid analysis if there is any suspicion of infection and radiography to see whether there is any remodelling of the extensor carpi radialis groove on the dorsodistal radius. Ultrasonography will determine if there is damage to the tendon *per se*, synovial proliferation or adhesion formation.
(c) The presence of lameness as a result of infection, or damage to the extensor carpi radialis tendon in association with new bone on the distal aspect of the radius, will lead to a poor-to-guarded prognosis.

107 Rectal tears are a rare but real hazard when pelvic or abdominal exploration is carried out by this route. The incidence is said to be higher in male horses than mares, possibly because they are more used to being examined in this manner. Alternative explanations are that the male has an inherent weakness in the rectum, or that examinations are carried out in males for reasons (colic or the location of an abdominal testis) that require palpation further into the abdomen than routine gynaecological examination of the mare.

The most common site for rectal damage is about 30 cm cranial to the anus and dorsally, i.e. longitudinally along the mesorectal attachment. This trauma may then cause haemorrhage (usually non-fatal) and escape of rectal contents into the peritoneal cavity. Fatal peritonitis is a common sequela.

It is often caused by experienced clinicians and is often unrecognised. In many cases, blood which is seen on the arm after examination of a horse per rectum is due to inconsequential superficial trauma. When tears do occur, the natural assumption of the examiner is that his/her fingers have penetrated the rectum and unless he/she is aware of the likely dorsal location of the lesion, re-examination will not be diagnostic.

Many factors that may contribute to rectal tears are not controllable so that it is impossible to give advice as to how they may be avoided. Since routine tranquillization of all horses and the complete elimination of external stimuli and peristalsis are not practical or possible, accidents can always occur. Advice to resist peristaltic contractions is unrealistic, although a gentle, relaxed and patient approach should always be advocated. Examinations should be terminated if the horse strains forcefully.

108 (a) Oxyuriasis due to infection with the pinworm *Oxyuris equi.*
(b) Perineal pruritus leads to self-trauma of the tailhead or hindquarters on stable fittings, fencing, etc. It is thought that the process of egg laying by the adult worms as they emerge through the anus causes irritation of the adjacent skin.
(c) The distribution of the skin lesions is suggestive of oxyuriasis. Sweet itch may give rise to similar lesions but in that condition there are usually also lesions present in the mane and withers. The presence of streaks of sticky, grey/yellow material in the perineum is indicative of oxyuriasis, and microscopic identification of typical, operculate, flat-sided, *O. equi* eggs in this material will confirm the diagnosis.
(d) Broad-spectrum anthelmintic. Cleaning the perineal skin with a cloth will reduce further contamination of the environment with oxyuris eggs.

109 (a) *Senecio jacobaea* (common ragwort). The toxic principles are the pyrrolizidine alkaloids.
(b) The section shows loss of hepatocytes and replacement with fibrous tissue (*Figure 280*). Several megalocytes (abnormally large hepatocytes) are visible. These findings are

typical of ragwort poisoning, although similar changes occur in aflatoxicosis.

(c) Pyrrolizidine alkaloids are metabolised to highly toxic pyrroles which have an antimitotic effect resulting in megalocytosis. Fibrosis occurs in response to parenchymal degeneration.

(d) Serum gamma glutamyl transferase (GGT) is the most sensitive indicator of liver damage in subclinical ragwort poisoning.

110 (a) Diabetes mellitus (DM). DM is defined as a persistent hyperglycaemia due to a relative or absolute deficiency of insulin. In the horse, true DM has not been convincingly documented and most cases occur in association with another disease state. Although DM occurs uncommonly in the horse it is often detected in cases of Cushing's disease due to pituitary adenoma.

(b) This pony is only 4 years old and, except for increased thirst and weight loss, is exhibiting none of the signs of hyperadrenocorticism of Cushing's disease. The most likely cause of DM in this pony is chronic pancreatitis, which is usually considered to result from migration of strongyle larvae, particularly *Strongylus equinus*.

(c) Further investigation should be directed towards study of glucose metabolism and identification of an underlying cause.

Horses with DM would, by definition, have resting hyperglycaemia, and following intravenous glucose loading there would be prolonged duration of the induced hyperglycaemia. It would be useful to measure plasma glucose levels following administration of intravenous regular insulin: if plasma glucose levels are not lowered then this would confirm insulin resistance as the mechanism of DM, rather than deficient insulin production which is assumed in pancreatitis.

Confirmation of pancreatitis would require measurement of levels of lipase and amylase in plasma and peritoneal fluid. Equine pancreas contains high concentrations of gamma glutamyl transferase (GGT) such that cases of equine DM may have raised plasma GGT levels.

111 (a) The exposed bone is devitalised and has lost its periosteal covering. It will sequestrate and eventually slough.

(b) Surgically remove the devitalised bone.

(c) There will probably be granulation tissue present under the necrotic bone and this will expand and fill the area immediately the bone is removed. Healing should then progress without further complication. Casting the limb may prevent the development of exuberant granulation tissue.

112 (a) There are several strongyle eggs in the faecal matter.

(b) The number of eggs and the identification of the species of worm are important. Cyathostome and strongylus species eggs are very similar but can be differentiated by artificial hatching and identification of the larvae. The level of infestation in in-contact horses should be determined.

(c) Resistance to fenbendazole and related anthelmintics is known to exist and the owner should regularly check on the efficacy of the anthelmintic regimen. All horses sharing pasture should be treated similarly (by regular post-treatment worm egg counts). Tremendous benefits may be accrued from removal of faeces from pasture. The timing of anthelmintic treatments and the drug used should be reappraised. Grazing hygiene should be maintained as far as practicable.

113 (a) See *Figure 281:* proper ligament of the testes – elongated in the incomplete abdominally retained testis (1); tail of the epididymis (2); ligament of the tail of the epididymis (3); vaginal process (4).

(b)
- Temporary inguinal retention.
- Permanent inguinal retention.
- Incomplete abdominal retention.
- Complete abdominal retention.
- Unilateral or bilateral.

(c)
- *Oestrone sulphate test* – In horses over 3 years old a single blood sample can be assayed for oestrone sulphate: geldings less than 100 pg/ml; cryptorchids more than 400 pg/ml.
- *Testosterone stimulation test* – In horses under 3 years old and donkeys of any age. Serum testosterone concentrations are assayed before and 30 min to 2 h post-stimulation with 6000 iu human chorionic gonadotrophin. Cryptorchids have a testosterone concentration of greater than 100 pg/ml before and a higher level following stimulation.

114 (a) This case would probably be classified as 'idiopathic chronic diarrhoea'. No specific diagnosis can be reached in up to 50% of cases of chronic diarrhoea. Potential mechanisms that may be important in such cases include abnormalities of fermentation, secretion or motility in the caecum and/or colon.

(b) Multiple bowel wall biopsies (obtained via laparotomy) are valuable in the diagnosis of some cases of chronic diarrhoea, but in cases where functional abnormalities are involved, this is unlikely to yield any useful information.

(c) There are many treatments that may be tried in such cases. These include dietary manipulation (some cases improve when kept on grass, others when kept on dry feed), intestinal absorbents and protectants (kaolin, powdered chalk, bismuth subsalicylate, etc.), transfaunation with fresh caecal contents or faecal liquor, chloro-iodo-hydroxy-quinoline, codeine phosphate, phenoxybenzamine, probiotics, etc.

115 (a) Hydatid cysts. Large fluid-filled cysts with a heavy fibrous capsule are present on the surface of this liver. Some animals will have multiple, small cysts throughout the liver parenchyma and cysts are occasionally found in other organs. The cysts contain the larval stages of the canine tapeworm *Echinococcus granulosus equinus* for which the horse is an intermediate host.

(b) Even in cases such as the one illustrated, in which a large proportion of the liver is involved in the hydatid lesions, the condition appears to be of little pathogenic significance to the horse.

(c) Hydatid cysts in horses have no zoonotic significance since *E. g. equinus* has an exclusively canine–equine cycle and has never been identified in other animals.

116 (a) These horses are probably affected by a contagious respiratory disease, which is most likely viral in nature. The majority of horses that suddenly start coughing are suffering from an upper respiratory tract viral infection. A number of different viruses can be involved in such cases, including equine influenza, equine herpesvirus, equine rhinovirus, etc. A viral cause should not be discounted in a vaccinated horse; even horses vaccinated against influenza can become infected by that virus (especially if the vaccination was performed more than 6 months previously), although the severity of the disease is generally less than in unvaccinated and non-immune animals. Confirmation of the nature of the virus infection requires virus isolation and/or serological techniques, but these investigations are usually not necessary.

(b) Specific therapy of horses with viral infections is often not required. The most important consideration in their management is rest until full recovery has taken place (usually 7–14 days in mild infections). Viral infections are a common predisposing factor in the development of airway hypersensitivity (i.e. COPD), and attempts should be made to reduce the exposure of infected horses to environmental antigens (primarily hay and straw dusts). Symptomatic therapy with bronchodilators (e.g. clenbuterol) and/or mucolytics can help speed the resolution of clinical disease. Antibiotic therapy is unnecessary unless severe secondary bacterial infections are suspected. Non-steroidal anti-inflammatory agents can also be beneficial in severe infections (i.e. where there is a high and prolonged fever or anorexia).

117 (a) The most likely cause of the murmur is a ventricular septal defect, with blood shunting from the left to the right ventricle. Tricuspid regurgitation would also result in a systolic murmur with its point of maximum intensity over the tricuspid valve; however, even in very severe cases, these murmurs tend not to radiate ventrally along the sternal border. It may be that this pony has tricuspid regurgitation and a ventricular septal defect.

(b) The image shows left atrial dilatation due to volume overload of the left side of the heart. The right side of the heart is also dilated with the septum pushed across towards the left ventricle. As this is a systolic frame it suggests that the horse has pulmonary hypertension with elevated right ventricular pressures. This would also account for the increased intensity of the second heart sound. If a ventricular septal defect is present it is likely to be a large defect with significant volume flow.

(c) Ventricular septal defects are most commonly located in the membranous septum underneath the right coronary cusp of the aortic valve and the septal leaflet of the tricuspid valve. Careful investigation of this area would be necessary to confirm the diagnosis of a ventricular septal defect in a case with a murmur of this type. The echocardiogram in *Figure 282* was obtained from the same pony. The transducer has been rotated slightly and angled cranially to image the aorta (AO). The ventricular septal defect (VSD) can now be seen clearly.

(d) This pony is already showing signs of left-sided volume overload. This will probably result in an increase in the left ventricular end diastolic pressure. Dilatation of the left ventricle will occur with stretching of the mitral valve annulus leading to mitral regurgitation. This will add to the volume overload of the left atrium resulting in elevated left atrial pressures and pulmonary congestion. Congestive cardiac failure will develop. Increased blood flow through the pulmonary circulation due to the left-to-right shunt will lead to pulmonary hypertension and elevated right ventricular systolic pressures. The right ventricle is not designed as a high-pressure pump, and although hypertrophy will occur the ventricle will ultimately dilate. Ventricular dilatation will result in malposition of the papillary muscles and stretching of the valve annulus, leading to tricuspid regurgitation. Severe tricuspid regurgitation will result in an increase in right atrial and systemic venous pressure, resulting in congestion. Reverse or bidirectional shunting will occur as ventricular pressures rise. Thus the prognosis is poor.

118 See *Figure 283*.
(a) Acute; there is no evidence of adjacent articular degeneration, remodelling of osseous contour or periarticular osteophyte formation, and there is little synovial proliferation.
(b) Dorsolateral–palmaromedial oblique and flexed lateromedial projections most consistently predict the presence of chip fractures in this location.

119 (a) The plant is *Senecio jacobaea* (ragwort) and the pyrrolizidine alkaloid it contains is a significant cause of poisoning in horses.
(b) Repeated or persistent ingestion of this plant is responsible for the development of a severe hepatic cirrhosis. The clinical signs may be limited to weight loss, hypoproteinaemia, ascites, photosensitisation and icterus but terminate in hepatoencephalopathy.
(c) The live plant is generally unpalatable to grazing horses and it is consumed only under conditions of starvation. Dead plants seem to be more palatable and, when included in hay, horses are unable to discriminate and significant ingestion may occur. All fields in which horses are grazed or which are cut for hay should be free of the plant. Plants should be pulled up entirely before the seeding season, and removed from the field.

120 The condition is known as suture or frontal periostitis and the diagnosis can be confirmed by a skyline radiograph of the lesion with the horse in the standing position (*Figure 284*). Both endosteal and periosteal new bone formation will be visible but the overall swelling far exceeds the bony reaction.
   The cause of suture periostitis is not known, although trauma is an obvious candidate. The most common site is along the line taken by the frontonasal suture. Most lesions are symmetrical about the midline but occasionally they are sufficiently extensive to compromise lacrimal flow.
   The behaviour of suture periostitis is comparable to 'splints' on the metacarpal bones in as much as they arise by elevation of the periosteum with subperiosteal haemorrhage which then ossifies. The initial soft-tissue response may be reduced by cold compresses and anti-inflammatory medication. Considerable bony modelling at the site will generally leave no more than a minor cosmetic blemish, but even this could be disastrous for a show horse. The bony reaction does not involve the nasal airways and respiratory obstruction is never a feature. However, a serous nasal discharge may be present in peracute cases.

121 (a) The laceration can easily be repaired. Sedate the horse (detomidine and butorphanol is a useful combination). Infiltrate the wound edges with a non-irritant local anaesthetic (e.g. 1% mepivacaine, without adrenaline). Thoroughly flush the wound first with liberal amounts of water and povidone-iodine or chlorhexidine.
   There may be significant swelling after suturing the wound, therefore it would be prudent to apply some tension sutures. Oppose the skin edges using a simple interrupted pattern with, for example, polypropylene.
(b) Yes, the wound is vertical, and the blood supply should not be compromised. It will drain well. There is not too much movement at this site and therefore dehiscence should not occur.
(c) No, since only skin and fascia have been injured.

122 (a) Congenital heart malformation with right-to-left shunt or severe pulmonary disease, such as severe pneumonia, atelectasis, pneumothorax, congenital malformation, etc.
(b) Radiograph the thorax and perform an ultrasonographic examination of the heart. Special cardiac examination may then be indicated (inject bubbles into right heart, chamber pressures, etc.). Measurement of complete blood count and fibrinogen may be indicated if pneumonia is suspected.

123 (a) The horse is anaemic, and has a leucocytosis and hyperfibrinogenaemia; these are probably the result of chronic infection/inflammation/neoplasia. The urea is mildly raised, and urine specific gravity is low. Serum calcium is significantly elevated.
(b) The cause of the hypercalcaemia and soft-tissue mineralisation was most likely to have been associated with the apparent neoplasia of the spleen (i.e. ectopic- or pseudo-hyperparathyroidism). Other possible causes would include primary hyperparathyroidism, widespread bone destruction, primary renal disease, vitamin D toxicosis or exposure to calcinogenic plants. Hypercalcaemic nephropathy results in the production of dilute urine of low specific gravity, with polyuria and polydipsia. Calcification of the endocardium and heart valves was the probable cause of the heart murmur. Ectopic hyperparathyroidism has been recorded in association with a number of different tumours in the horse, most commonly lymphosarcoma.

124 (a) Yes.
(b) Large, oval, pink disc with radiating fine retinal vessels and a clear tapetal fundus.

125 The laryngoscopic view illustrates a case of cricopharyngeal aplasia, sometimes known as rostral displacement of the palatal arch. This is an obvious case of a condition which arises through maldevelopment of derivatives of the fourth branchial arch. The common structures to be absent are:
- Cricopharyngeus muscles – the proximal oesophageal sphincter.
- Cricothyroid articulation.
- Caudal portion of thyroid lamina.
- Cricothyroideus muscles.

The absence of normal cricothyroid articulations compromises the mechanical effect of the laryngeal abductor muscles. This combined with the free caudal pillars of the arcus palatopharyngeus causes the abnormal respiratory noises.

Absence of an effective proximal oesophageal sphincter renders the horse an involuntary air swallower as the oesophagus is permanently open (*Figure 285*). Thus, other signs of this condition include:
- Audible eructation.
- Dysphagia with nasal discharge and coughing.
- Unthriftiness.
- Colic.

There is no remedy for this major congenital disorder.

126 (a) A fracture of the tuber coxae, iliac wing or shaft or possibly the pubis. Given the degree of asymmetry the latter is less likely.
(b) Rectal examination, and, if possible, standing radiography of the pelvis. [*Editor's Note*: This is a potentially dangerous procedure; radiography performed under a general anaesthesia is preferable, but must be delayed for some weeks after surgery.]
(c) If the injury involves the ilium, but not the acetabulum, the prognosis is rather better than if the injury is associated with disruption of the coxofemoral joint.

127 (a) Jaundice, petechial haemorrhages and a brownish-red colour at the gingival margin (the so-called toxic line sometimes seen in toxaemia).
(b) The history and clinical findings suggest equine hyperlipaemia.
(c) Examine the serum or plasma which usually appear opaque due to the presence of excessive quantities of lipids. Triglyceride assay of serum can be used to quantify the degree of lipaemia.
(d) Treatment involves restoration of a positive energy balance by providing high-energy foods and by glucose administration by stomach tube. As glucose uptake from the blood to the tissues is impaired, insulin therapy is indicated concurrently. Acidosis may occur, in which case sodium bicarbonate therapy is indicated. Induction of foaling or abortion may be considered, since this may improve the prognosis.
(e) Serum triglyceride levels should be monitored. GLDH and GGT are useful to follow resolution of fatty liver.

128 (a) Hypercalcaemic nephropathy. Mineralised casts can be seen within nephrons and collecting ducts (Von Kossa stain is selective for calcium). Other histopathological changes which were identified in the kidneys of this animal included tubular degeneration and foci of interstitial fibrosis.
(b)
• Mineralisation of soft tissues of other organs, e.g. heart and great vessels.
• Neoplasia.
• Hypercalcaemic nephropathy in the horse has been reported to occur as part of the paraneoplastic syndrome of pseudo-hyperparathyroidism. The pathogenesis of hypercalcaemia in this condition is considered to be the secretion of ectopic humoral substances (such as parathyroid hormone analogues, prostaglandin E2, vitamin D-like osteolytic sterols or osteoclast activating factor) by a non-endocrine tumour. In the horse pseudo-hyperparathyroidism has been found in association with lymphosarcoma, ovarian stromal tumours, gastric carcinoma, adrenocortical carcinoma and abdominal mesothelioma.
The case illustrated here had splenic lymphosarcoma which was palpable per rectum and which could be identified by ultrasonography.

129 (a) The earliest stage at which pregnancy can be detected by ultrasonography is 11 or 12 days after ovulation. If a mare has had a synchronous double ovulation then twins could be detected at that time. However, because many mares have double ovulations 24 or more hours apart, there is little practical point in scanning this early. At 14 days post-ovulation most twin conceptuses should be detectable. However, it is possible for ova to be fertilised 4 or more days apart. This is most likely to happen if:
• A second ovulation occurs early in dioestrus.
• The mare is covered after the first ovulation.
• The stallion has good-quality semen; this can often remain viable for 4 days or more.
(b) The earliest that pregnancy can be diagnosed conclusively by palpation is about 21 days after ovulation. This is usually easier in ponies than in horses and the technique requires practised skills. Twin pregnancies which are distributed bilaterally (one in each horn) can be detected at 21 days if ovulations occurred at the same time. However, if a longer interval occurred between ovulations, a bilateral twin pregnancy would not be easily diagnosed at this time. Unilateral twins, i.e. where both conceptuses develop together at the base of the same uterine horn, will always be palpated as a single pregnancy and, despite expectations, the palpable size of a twin pregnancy is not appreciably greater than a single.

130 (a) *Dermatophilus congolensis*; rain scald, mud fever.
(b)
● Scabs from fresh lesions.
● Impression smears from underneath a fresh scab; stain with new methylene blue or Giemsa.
(c) Microaerophilic, to prevent overgrowth by other skin contaminants.
(d)
● Penicillin 10 mg/kg and streptomycin 10 mg/kg given intramuscularly for 3–5 days.
● Daily washing with 5% potassium permanganate.
● Remove the horses from contact with wet grass and rain.

131 (a)
● Maxillary sinus – medial canthus of the orbit to the nasomaxillary notch, facial crest infraorbital foramen and ventral rim of orbit.
● Frontal sinus – medial canthus of the orbit to the nasomaxillary notch, sagittal midline and supraorbital process.
(b)
● Do not transect the line of the nasolacrimal duct (medial canthus of the orbit to the nasomaxillary notch).
● Ensure the base of the skin flap is twice the length of its depth.
● Preserve the periosteal margin.
● Discard or hinge back the bone flap, by fracturing it along its fourth side, preserving its periosteal attachments if it is to be retained.
● The animal's age dictates the amount of dental tissue remaining within the maxillary sinus and therefore the exposure and access to the ventral conchal sinus, medially.
● Haemorrhage may be controlled by direct compression or temporary bilateral caratoid artery occlusion. Use a well-inflated cuffed endotracheal tube and ensure a facility to lower the head below the level of the trachea during the intraoperative period. Intensive intraoperative fluid therapy is desirable.
● Postoperative irrigation of the paranasal sinuses must be facilitated.
(c)
● Postoperative haemorrhage – controlled by the intraoperative placement of a sock and bandage compression pack that is led out via the nares. This may be gradually removed over 72 h.
● Postoperative sinus drainage/irrigation – aggressive postoperative irrigation to the nares via an indwelling Foley balloon catheter, exiting separately from the primary incision line, will aid resolution of existing pathology and residual haematoma formation.
● Wound breakdown – a result of inadequate periosteal and skin closure (non-airtight seal), sequestra formation from fracture of the bone flap, or bone necrosis from thermal damage of the bone margin created by the air saw.

132 This is a normal foal with no compression of its cervical spinal cord (substantiated by histopathological evaluation). With young horses and firm flexion of the neck, the ventral dye columns and a substantial proportion of the dorsal dye columns can be obliterated or attenuated. In interpreting such a myelogram it is better to look at the minimum sagittal dimensions of the vertebral canal as well as the minimum sagittal diameters of the myelographic (dural) column and compare with normal values. In this case these values were well within the normal range for horses under 320 kg body weight.

133 A substantial number of mares lose well-established pregnancies either by early resorption or later abortion for undiagnosed reasons. Since it is well known that progesterone is the hormone essential for the maintenance of pregnancy, it appears logical to assume that some losses might be due to insufficient progesterone production. This possibility is supported by the fact that progesterone production in the mare depends on three sources. Initially the corpus luteum verum of pregnancy was thought to be active only until the fortieth day, although there is strong evidence that it does not regress at this time. After 40 days more luteal tissue is formed by further ovulations or luteinisations of unruptured follicles under the influence of eCG and pituitary FSH. Around 100 days the placenta (the actual site of synthesis is unknown) becomes responsible for progesterone production and there appears to be a gradual 'handover' from the regressing corpora lutea to the increasingly active placenta.

These changes influence plasma progesterone concentrations. That formed in the ovary must travel to the uterus via the general circulation, so that plasma values reflect luteal activity. However, particularly between the sixteenth and fortieth days, plasma progesterone concentrations may fall to around 1 ng/ml without any evidence of a threat to pregnancy well-being. Also after the rise in progesterone production between 40 and about 120 days, circulating values are usually also low because placental progesterone influences the myometrium and cervix without entering the circulation.

In mares known to have lost their pregnancies previously, progesterone therapy (implants, injections in oil, and more recently orally active synthetic progestagens) have been used empirically to prevent subsequent losses. Success must be interpreted cautiously because in most cases the circumstances of previous pregnancy failures are not known. However, because such treatment is not harmful many claims for their efficacy have been made, although these are undoubtedly exaggerated. No 'control' studies have been conducted in this area but, in particular, to claim that progesterone therapy prevents resorption (rather than abortion) is a contradiction in terms because this form of early pregnancy loss is, by definition, one that occurs whilst luteal function persists.

134 (a) Spasmodic colic.
(b)
- Antispasmolytic (i.e. hyoscine-N-butylbromide and dipyrone 20 ml/450 kg). This is usually enough to settle this type of colic.
- Analgesic. Phenylbutazone or xylazine may be necessary.
(c)
- Flunixin meglumine should not be used unless its antiendotoxic effect is required in the event of the case becoming surgical. If given early in a medical case it will mask signs of septic shock until too late should the case turn out to be surgical. (See *Figure 286*, which is an example of this.)
- Acetylpromazine is hypotensive. This will compromise a patient that develops endotoxic shock.
(d) Have all food removed and ensure that the horse cannot eat its bed, and allow water. Instruct the owner to observe the animal closely; telephone in 2 h for a progress report. If in doubt revisit. Do not leave it to the owner to ring you if worried. It is rarely possible to be sure at your first examination that you have a simple medical case. You will have a better idea 2 h later.

135 (a) Suturing could be accomplished by means of vertical mattress sutures and tension sutures, but wound breakdown is likely to occur due to movement and vertical tension and possible compromise of the blood supply to the distal flap.
(b) Moist areas and tension areas would appear after about 5–7 days, with wound dehiscence at approximately 10 days.
(c) Secondary intention healing.
(d) The initial treatment of choice depends partly on available finance. It is likely that if the wound is sutured at least part of it may break down, but some benefit may have been achieved. The initial wound will heal satisfactorily by second intention, albeit slowly.

136 (a) There is infiltration of the colon wall by polymorphonuclear leucocytes and mononuclear cells. There is submucosal oedema and necrosis of the mucosa.
(b) The colonic contents are likely to be foul smelling and dark brown or red. The surface of the colon would appear haemorrhagic; the mucosa may be sloughing.
(c) The clinical and post-mortem features indicate that the horse was affected by an acute colitis/enteritis, resulting in severe dehydration, toxaemia and death. Potential causes of this syndrome include acute salmonellosis, intestinal clostridiosis, colitis X, Potomac horse fever (equine monocytic ehrlichiosis), antibiotic-associated enteritis and non-steroidal anti-inflammatory drug toxicity. The first three conditions seem most likely in this case.
(d) The clinical and post-mortem features of all forms of acute colitides are similar. Differentiation between them relies on laboratory investigations. In particular, bacteriological culture of faeces and intestinal contents are essential to diagnose salmonellosis and clostridiosis; cultures from cases of colitis X yield normal bacterial flora only. Potomac horse fever is generally diagnosed serologically.

137 (a) A haemorrhagic discharge and a purulent discharge are visible at the ostia of the auditory tube diverticula (ATD) (guttural pouches).
(b) The presence of blood issuing from the ATD may be a sign of impending or existent erosion of the internal carotid artery in cases of ATD mycosis. In this case it is unlikely that such a lesion is present since it is not usually also associated with a purulent discharge, but further examinations should be undertaken to identify the cause of the bleeding.
(c) In view of the presence of a purulent discharge at the other ostium it is likely that this horse has suffered from a ruptured pharyngeal abscess with consequent haemorrhage. Such complications are commonly encountered following *Streptococcus equi* infections.

138 (a) Thiopentone sodium, guaphenesin or chloral hydrate. These are highly irritant substances if injected perivascularly.
(b)
- In equine anaesthesia, highly concentrated solutions (5–15%) of these drugs are used. Known or suspected perivascular injection of chemically irritant substances should be treated immediately by dilution with an isotonic physiological solution, e.g. Hartmann's solution. Hyaluronidase and local anaesthetic (without adrenaline) may be incorporated into this treatment regimen.
- The exact time-course of each case differs, but symptomatic treatment of the inflammatory response using systemic non-steroidal anti-inflammatory drugs and topical application of hyaluronidase ointment or a desloughing agent is indicated and will reduce discomfort. In severe cases, with extensive areas of thrombosis and tissue

necrosis, as illustrated here, surgical drainage and debridement are the treatments of choice once the initial inflammatory response has subsided.
(c) The risk of perivascular injection of such drugs is minimised if a jugular vein catheter is employed, rather than injection via a needle.

139 Refer to *Figure 287*.
(a) This is a non-marginal osteochondral effect. These have been referred to as incomplete slab fractures of the third carpal bone.
(b) A flexed dorsoproximal–dorsodistal oblique projection. With the carpus flexed to produce a horizontal position of the metacarpus a beam angle of approximately 30° to the horizontal is usually employed (flexed D30°Pr-DDiO).
(c) The extensor carpi radialis tendon and its synovial sheath. Surgical approaches to this area (arthroscopic or by arthrotomy) are therefore directed medial to this structure.

140 Assessment of haematological changes, serum protein, urea, creatinine, electrolytes and acid–base balance would be of value in the management of a case like this. The resultant fluid and electrolyte loss necessitates intravenous fluid administration, and correction of metabolic acidosis is likely to be necessary.

Sodium and chloride deficits can be measured with acceptable accuracy because these electrolytes are extracellular. The level of deficit can be measured from the following formula:

[Normal Na^+ (mmol/l) − measured Na^+ (mmol/l) × body weight (kg)/3] = Na^+ deficit (mmol/l)

Potassium deficits are more difficult to assess because this ion is primarily intracellular. As a result, measurement of serum or plasma potassium levels does not effectively reflect total body potassium status. However, in general low K^+ values (<2.5 mmol/l) may indicate a significant K^+ deficit.

Multi-electrolyte solutions are therefore preferable to normal saline. Large volumes of fluids, perhaps 20–50 litres, may be required in cases of colitis, and if severe shock develops high flow rates of up to 10 l/h may be required. The volume of selected replacement fluid can be calculated from the following formula:

Electrolyte deficit (mmol/l) − concentration of electrolyte in replacement fluid (mmol/l) = volume of replacement fluid (l) needed to correct estimated electrolyte deficit

Hydration status can be assessed by monitoring both PCV and serum or plasma proteins. Both of these haematological and blood biochemical parameters should be monitored concurrently. Although either may reflect dehydration, a fall in protein levels can occur when the PCV is rising, and this divergence can reflect endotoxaemia.

The principal acid–base disturbance is metabolic acidosis and this can be monitored through measurement of bicarbonate values from arterial blood gas estimations. In general, bicarbonate values of <15 mmol/l necessitate intravenous bicarbonate administration. Bicarbonate should not be administered rapidly (one-half to two-thirds of the deficit can be replaced in half an hour, the remainder over several hours), nor, in general, other than as a 5% solution.

141 (a) Dorsopalmar, dorsolateral–palmaromedial oblique, dorsomedial–palmarolateral oblique and lateromedial (and/or flexed lateromedial) views.
(b) There is a small well-rounded mineralised opacity or body on the proximal aspect of the proximal phalanx. There is a suggestion of a small lucent defect in the proximodorsal aspect of the proximal phalanx distal to the mineralised body.
(c) Intra-articular analgesia of the metacarpophalangeal joint should substantially improve the lameness. Such mineralised pieces can occur unilaterally or bilaterally and may be insignificant incidental findings.
(d)
- Separate centre of ossification.
- Manifestation of osteochondrosis.
- Old chip fracture.
- Mineralisation in the joint capsule.

(e) Surgical removal of the piece, preferably arthroscopically. This technique allows better appraisal of the joint than via an arthrotomy; it should be less traumatic and allows a shorter convalescence, with less risk of periarticular fibrosis.
(f) Fair to good depending on the presence or absence of other intra-articular pathology.

142 There is no cause for concern. You should check the mating date and the calculated pregnancy length, although the owner will usually have done this several times.
   Pregnancy length is normally very variable in the mare; if it is long, it usually means that the fetus is not developing at an optimal rate because of:
- Poor nutrition.
- Systemic disease in the mare.
- Extensive endometrial lesions reducing the effective placental area.
- Death of a twin followed by continuation of the pregnancy; growth of the viable fetus would have been initially slow because of competition for nutrition by the twin.

The owner's unfounded worries about the long gestation are usually:
- That a large foal will eventually be born and will cause dystocia. This will not happen. Even after gestation lengths of over 1 year the foal may be small due to the reasons previously given.
- That the foal is dead. This is also extremely unlikely because death of a foal causes a rapid fall in progesterone production (by the feto–maternal unit) and rapid expulsion (abortion). Therefore, mares do not retain dead single foals *in utero*. Rectal examination of the mare to elicit fetal movement may reassure an owner.

Induction of parturition should be avoided where possible because:
- If the mare does not foal soon after the administration of oxytocin or prostaglandin the clinician may have to spend many hours in close attendance. This is often uneconomical.
- An induced foal may be immature or dysmature and fail to survive.
- Dystocia may occur due to failure of the immature foal to assume the normal posture and position for birth.

143 (a) The horse has an abnormally long hair coat (hirsutism) for the time of year. The hair looks curly. The most common cause is a pituitary adenoma, in the pars intermedia.
(b) Common clinical signs include polydipsia/polyuria, diarrhoea, weight loss, colic and laminitis. Oestrus cycles may be suppressed or abnormal. Horses become more susceptible to concurrent diseases, especially infections.

(c) The disorder is generally slowly progressive. There is no known effective treatment, although cyproheptadine has been used to control clinical signs in mild cases.
(d) No, not directly. Although a high worm burden may be encountered as an incidental finding it is occasionally exceptionally high in these cases.

144 (a) Pythiosis (or phycomycosis).
(b)
- Streptococci and *Staphylococcus aureus* have been isolated from similar lesions.
- Subcutaneous mycotic infections are frequently pruritic as well as painful, whereas both streptococcal and staphylococcal infections are painful but not itchy.
- While not typical, lesions due to *Habronema* can infect this area also.
(c)
- Careful surgical excision.
- Followed by sodium iodide given intravenously at the rate of 1 g/15 kg body weight.
- Pack wound with amphotericin B daily.
- Systemic amphotericin B is also recommended in severe infections.

145 (a) Dorsopalmar, dorsolateral–palmaromedial oblique, palmarolateral–dorsomedial oblique, flexed lateromedial and dorsoproximal–dorsodistal oblique views.
(b) The dorsolateral–palmaromedial oblique view is shown in *Figures 116A* and *B*. The dorsoproximal–dorsodistal oblique view of the distal row of carpal bones is shown in *Figure 116C*.
(c) There is alteration in the trabecular pattern in the subchondral bone of the proximal articular surface of the third carpal bone in *Figures 116A* and *B*. In *Figure 116C* there is an incomplete sagittal fracture of the third carpal bone, and some medullary sclerosis involving the radial facet of the third carpal bone. (Compare the trabecular pattern with that of the second and fourth carpal bones.)
(d) Treatment: box rest (3 months); re-evaluate radiographically.
Prognosis: fair.

146 (a) There is enlargement on the medial aspect of the right hock, probably related to degenerative joint disease of one or more of the centrodistal (distal intertarsal) and tarsometatarsal joints (bone spavin). In this case the animal had degenerative joint disease affecting both joints.
(b) Such an animal may or may not be lame. In this case the animal had been slightly lame two years before but this had disappeared about 18 months before this picture was taken. The lameness on the left forelimb was the result of degenerative joint disease of the antebrachiocarpal (radiocarpal) joint.

147 (a)
- Elevated heart rate 90 beats/min.
- Elevated end diastolic pressures.
- No evidence of P-waves on the ECG or A-waves on the atrial trace.
- The left atrial trace shows large V-waves.
- Irregular ventricular rhythm.
- Low left ventricular systolic pressures.
(b) The large V-waves are indicative of mitral regurgitation. The left atrium is being filled in systole with blood from the pulmonary veins and with blood leaking through the mitral valve from the left ventricle. The regurgitation will cause elevated end

diastolic pressures and lead to a decrease in the cardiac output. The regurgitation will also result in stretching of the left atrium, predisposing the horse to atrial fibrillation.
(c) This horse will be showing signs associated with low cardiac output, exercise intolerance, weakness, depression, pale mucous membranes and cold extremities. It will also be showing signs of congestive cardiac failure, pulmonary oedema and dyspnoea due to the elevated left atrial pressures. If right-sided heart failure develops, signs of systemic venous congestion will become evident – subcutaneous oedema, pleural effusion and ascites.

148 (a) All four approaches have their indications.
- The ventral midline incision is the approach of choice for surgical exploration of a colic case. It gives the greatest single incision exposure of the peritoneal cavity and is the quickest approach. No major vessels, nerves or muscles are involved and it can be extended easily.
- The paramedian laparotomy is useful for cystotomy in the male patient.
- Flank incisions provide exposure to the base of the caecum and duodenum and have been used for the removal of enteroliths and the management of uterine torsions.
- The inguinal approach is performed for cryptorchidectomy and inguinal hernia repair.

(b) The most extensive exploration of the peritoneal cavity is achieved through a midline incision that starts over the umbilicus and extends sufficiently cranially (20 cm) to enable the surgeon to insert one arm for exploration. The short exploratory incision can be extended in either direction to accommodate any problem encountered. The more cranial the incision, the greater the risk for herniation; therefore the incision is placed as far caudally as possible. A post-umbilical approach is used for resections of the caudal portion of the small colon and for colorectostomy.
(c) The linea alba is incised carefully to avoid divergence from the midline, which would result in entry into the rectus abdominis muscle, particularly in the cranial portion of the incision. Incising only the linea alba will ensure easier closure and less chance of healing problems (herniation) at the incision site.
(d) The caecum is an important landmark, because it can be easily located and exteriorised and provides a good starting point for location of both the large and small intestine (*Figure 288*). The dorsal band of the caecum (arrowed) can be traced to the thin ileocaecal fold which continues into the antimesenteric band of the ileum. Once the ileum is located the small intestine can be examined systematically by moving proximad along the entire length of the jejunum. The lateral band of the caecum (arrowed) is continuous with the caecocolic fold which leads into the right ventral portion of the large colon. From this point the large colon can be explored.

If the caecum cannot be located a caecal or caecocolic intussusception or a complete torsion of the colon and caecum must be present.
(e)
- A separate closure of the *peritoneum* is not necessary but it helps to keep the bowel in a position to minimise accidental perforation during closure. It is also useful if there has been intraperitoneal soilage or intestinal resection and anastomosis. Closure is performed with a simple continuous suture of no. 1 polyglactin 910 (Vicryl) on a round-bodied needle.
- The *linea alba* is closed with a simple interrupted or a simple continuous pattern. Bites in the linea alba should be placed 1 cm apart. Double strands of no. 2 polyglycolic acid (Dexon) on a round-bodied needle are used. Polyglycolic acid has adequate strength for a sufficient length of time to allow healing to occur. It is

absorbable and so greatly reduces the risk of suture sinus formation.
- The *subcutaneous tissue* is closed with a continuous mattress layer of no. 1 polyglactin 910 (Vicryl). The main purpose of this layer is to cover the previous layer of sutures.
- The *skin* is closed with simple interrupted sutures or an interlocking continuous suture of a non-absorbable material such as no. 3 monofilament nylon or polymerised coprolactam (Supramid).

149 (a) The pupil is dilated. There is detachment of the retina.
(b) Yes, detachment of the retina and consequent 'light hunger' mydriasis may follow trauma and falls.
(c) Posterior uveitis and equine herpesvirus infection are possible factors, particularly when these are accompanied by chorioretinitis and vitrioretinal adhesions.
(d) If the condition is unilateral the prognosis for the animal is fair, but it is unlikely that sight will be restored in this eye. There are a number of top-class performance horses which have performed well despite only sight in one eye. Some horses do adopt a slightly abnormal head posture.

150 Occasionally a stallion or 'riggy' gelding is seen to cover a mare which is not intended for breeding. More rarely a mare may be covered by the wrong stallion at stud.

Unless and until it is safe to do so, the two horses should not be parted. The strategy is to allow the mare to ovulate and then cause luteolysis with prostaglandin, 6 or more days later. However, because mare owners instinctively expect that rapid treatment is most likely to succeed (uterine lavage and oestrogen injections are not effective) it may be difficult to get them to accept the delay in treatment.

In reality, giving prostaglandin 10 days or more after the mare is said to have gone out of oestrus should ensure that she then has a corpus luteum that is mature enough to be lysed by the treatment.

151 (a)
- Trephine and repulsion.
- Sinus bone flap and repulsion.
- Buccotomy and lateral alveolar wall resection.

(b)
- Trephine – simple approach, minimum of instrumentation, reduced anaesthetic time, allows postoperative management of alveolar socket.
- Sinus bone flap – increased intraoperative exposure, improved cosmetic results.
- Buccotomy and lateral wall resection – improved assurance of complete removal of dental tissue, paranasal sinus is not entered, but increased operating time and more accurate surgical approach required.

(c) Orosinus and orofacial fistulae, dental and bone sequestration, damage to adjacent dental radicles, fractured jaw.

152 The consequence of pregnancy failure in the mare depends on the stage of gestation at which it occurs. A small number of mares diagnosed as pregnant by ultrasound before the fifteenth day will subsequently return to oestrus and the conceptus will be expelled through the relaxed cervix. In these cases there is a failure to prevent luteolysis, probably because the conceptus does not 'inform' the endometrium of its presence, possibly due to a developmental anomaly.

Death of the conceptus during the time when the pregnancy is maintained by ovarian-derived progesterone, i.e. 15 to around 140 days, is not usually followed by immediate expulsion, because luteal activity persists and therefore circulating progesterone concentrations remain high. The dead conceptus (embryo or fetus) becomes autolysed *in utero* and dehydrated. This results in absorption of the fetal fluids and mummification of the embryo/fetus: the process has come to be known as resorption. Eventually, after natural regression of corpora lutea, the mare will come into oestrus, at which time the 'resorbed' conceptus is expelled but is rarely recovered; resorption could be said to be a form of mummification but because the dehydrated embryo/fetus has no skeleton, the expelled tissue is largely unrecognisable.

Somewhere between 120 and 150 days the placenta becomes responsible for producing the progesterone that maintains the pregnancy after the corpora lutea have regressed. The exact site of progesterone production has not been determined but precursors are undoubtedly formed in the fetus, probably in the endocrinologically active gonads. Therefore, if fetal death occurs at this stage of gestation, the progesterone influence in the uterus and cervix rapidly diminishes and the fetus is promptly aborted, i.e. mummification cannot occur.

Twin pregnancies can be an exception. Usually at this later stage of pregnancy, death of one fetus reduces endocrine control of the pregnancy sufficiently to cause abortion of the whole uterine contents, i.e. a slightly autolysed fetus and a fresh/viable fetus (*Figure 289A*). Occasionally, however, the pregnancy persists and the fetus that dies becomes dehydrated *in utero* (mummified) (*Figure 289B*); gestation is usually 'prolonged' and the live fetus may or may not be viable at birth.

153 (a) Not immediately because there is too much contamination, oedema and tissue damage.
(b)
• Debride all necrotic or devitalised tissue but leave as much skin as possible.
• Thoroughly clean the wound with non-irritant dressing such as 0.1% povidone-iodine. Apply bandage.
• Hose the wound daily and rebandage after dressing with 0.1% povidone-iodine.
• Take care to continue to fold skin flaps into the correct position before bandaging.
(c) Yes. Since the carpal joints have not been penetrated, healing should occur with minimal loss of function, despite severance of the extensor tendons. A slight change in gait may result due to this. There will ultimately be some scar tissue over the dorsal aspect of the carpus which may restrict flexion of the carpus, but is unlikely to be of any functional importance.

154 Refer to *Figure 290*.
(A) Plain swabs can be used for preparation of cervico-endometrial smears ((b) in question). These smears can be prepared by rolling the swab along a glass slide and then fixing the smear with a proprietary aerosol fixative prior to submission to the laboratory.
(B) The thin-wire-mounted swab is suitable for insertion into the clitoral sinus and fossa ((d) in question).
(C) The plastic-mounted swab is suitable for obtaining bacteria from the prepuce, the urethral fossa, the urethra and the pre-ejaculatory secretions of a stallion ((a) in question).

(D) The guarded swab is suitable for obtaining bacteria from the nasopharyngeal area in suspected cases of *Streptococcus equi* infection ((e) in question).

(E) The wire-mounted gauze swab is suitable for obtaining virus particles from the upper respiratory tract ((c) in question).

Swabs B, C and D should be placed in Amies transport medium on collection, prior to shipment to the laboratory. Swab E should be placed in cool virology transport medium and kept cool until delivered to the virology laboratory.

155 (a) Sodium penicillin (20 000–40 000 iu/kg q.i.d.) is often used intravenously for 3 days. If contamination has occurred during surgery, gentamycin (2.2 g/kg t.i.d.), kanamycin (5 mg/kg t.i.d.) or neomycin (6.75 mg/kg t.i.d.) can be added to the penicillin regimen and continued for up to 5 days postoperatively.

Overlong use of antibiotics is unnecessary because:

- The determining factor in postoperative infections is the presence of viable organisms in the surgical site at the time of wound closure.
- Antibiotics poorly penetrate the wound once it is sealed with fibrin.
- Prolonged use increases the risk of nosocomial infections and/or drug-potentiated salmonellosis.

(b) Recommendations on early feeding and watering in the postoperative patient vary widely, according to the subjective assessment of how this affects the return of gut peristalsis.

In the author's practice, water can be offered in small amounts (2 l) from 2 h postoperatively, if no evidence of gastric dilatation is found at surgery and the horse appears comfortable after recovery. After 12 h water is offered ad lib.

Provided evidence of gut motility is present, small amounts of grass or hay can be fed from 12 h postoperatively. If this is followed by normal defaecation the horse can be fed bran mashes from 24 h onwards. If intestinal transit is well established by the third day after surgery, the animal is gradually returned to full feed and ad lib hay over the next 5 days.

Water and food should be withheld immediately if any suggestion of impending ileus is present (absence of borborygmi and defaecation, gastric reflux).

(c) Skin sutures should be removed from abdominal incisions at 2 weeks in uncomplicated cases. This can be done by removing alternating sutures on a first visit and taking out the remaining sutures 2 days later.

(d) The animal should be confined to a box for a period of 3 months. Daily handwalking is advisable to control the common occurrence of ventral peri-incisional oedema, to fight boredom and to maintain some level of fitness. Any other form of exercise or free access to a paddock is unacceptable since the disruptive forces generated by playful paddock behaviour can result in herniation at the incision site.

(e) The horse can usually be returned to a normal feeding routine 1–2 weeks after surgery. It should not be fed excessive amounts of energy or protein, something many horse owners wrongly assume during convalescence from abdominal surgery. A 'non-heating' diet with plenty of hay will help to ensure that the animal is manageable both in the stable and during hand-walking sessions.

156 (a) Pale mucous membranes, epistaxis, petechial haemorrhage, hindlimb oedema with a sharply defined 'cut-off'.

(b) Purpura haemorrhagica, idiopathic or drug-induced thrombocytopenic purpura, disseminated intravascular coagulopathy (DIC). Other diseases resulting in a vasculitis include African horse sickness and equine viral arteritis. In view of the preceding history of an upper respiratory tract infection, purpura haemorrhagica is the most likely clinical diagnosis.

(c) Cases of purpura haemorrhagica often have a history of a viral or bacterial (streptococcal) infection in the previous 3–5 weeks. Thrombocytopenic conditions are rare and may arise following the administration of platelet-suppressing drugs or from autoimmune platelet destruction. DIC is most often associated with toxaemic or septicaemic disorders.

(d) Anaemia is a common, non-diagnostic feature. Blood samples are generally unhelpful in cases of purpura haemorrhagica, with platelet counts and clotting parameters usually normal. There may be non-specific neutrophilia. Bone marrow biopsy will reveal a regenerative myeloid : erythroid ratio. Idiopathic or drug-induced thrombocytopenia is associated with thrombocytopenia (<40 000/μl) and prolonged bleeding time. DIC is frequently associated with a non-specific leucocytosis and neutrophilia, with or without a leftward shift and elevated fibrinogen.

157 (a) Partial cataract.
(b) A dark iris denoting an associated uveitis, a small corneal scar at 7 o'clock and some irregularity in the corneal reflection.
(c) Significant abnormalities of this eye and defective vision on this side.

158 (a) The most likely respiratory cause of poor performance in this horse is low grade chronic obstructive pulmonary disease (COPD). This disease results from a sensitivity to inhaled dusts (primarily mould spores associated with hay and straw dusts).
(b) The most valuable diagnostic tests to confirm the presence of COPD are endoscopic examination of the lower airways, and cytological examination of samples of lower airway secretions obtained by lavage. Endoscopy may reveal a lower airway discharge (which frequently pools in the trachea at the level of the thoracic inlet), or inflammation/oedema of the bronchial walls. Samples of secretions for cytological examination may be obtained from the trachea (tracheal wash) or from the more distal airways (bronchoalveolar lavage); the latter is the preferred technique in cases of diffuse lung disease such as COPD where the major site of pathology is in the small airways (bronchioles). A neutrophilia in the secretions is expected in cases of COPD. Pulmonary function tests (e.g. intrapleural pressure measurement) and arterial blood gas analysis can be helpful if the facilities to perform these tests are available.

159 (a) Recurrent haemarthrosis. Lameness is usually sudden in onset during or after exercise, and may be very severe. It generally decreases markedly within the following 24–48 h. Arthrocentesis and removal of haemorrhage can produce rapid relief of acute severe pain.
(b) Synoviocentesis following exercise may demonstrate the recurrent nature of the pathology. Blood clotting studies will help determine a local or systemic problem, and further information may be determined from synovial biopsy (*Figure 291*).

160 (a) There is a smoothly outlined, approximately oval-shaped osseous body, with a suggestion of cortical and medullary structure, on the cranial aspect of the patella. This osseous body is likely to be of long standing. There is a well-defined small notch in the apex (distal aspect) of the patella. There is a suggestion of flattening of the middle one-third of the lateral trochlear ridge of the femur.

(b) Caudocranial, additional caudolateral–craniomedial oblique views, a flexed lateromedial view and a cranioproximal–craniodistal oblique view. These should permit the exclusion of other concurrent abnormalities; it is important to exclude a fracture of the patella, a common event horse injury, which may only be detectable in a cranioproximal–craniodistal oblique view. Additional oblique views should enable better assessment of the trochlear ridges. A flexed lateromedial view is helpful both to determine whether the fragment is mobile (*Figure 292*) and to assess better the proximal aspect of the lateral trochlear ridge of the femur and also the proximal tibia in the region of insertion of the cranial cruciate ligament.
(c) The osseous body may have arisen secondarily to osteochondrosis of the lateral trochlear ridge of the femur. Detached osteochondral fragments may enlarge progressively. Such bodies may sit immobile, innocuously within a joint, but if they become mobile they are likely to cause lameness.
(d) Surgical removal of the fragment. (Highly mobile fragments may be difficult to retrieve arthroscopically since they may move considerably when the joint has been inflated prior to insertion of the arthroscope, and thereafter. Arthrotomy may be the method of choice.) The prognosis is good.

161 (a) The moderately raised PCV, total protein, blood urea and alkaline phosphatase are consistent with dehydration. The latter has not reached the levels sometimes seen in colic associated with ischaemia of the gut. Plasma cortisol is usually markedly raised in grass sickness, exceeding the values attributable to stress alone.
(b) Serum haptoglobin increases three- to five-fold in acute grass sickness. Peritoneal fluid is yellow but has a high protein content comparable with that of ischaemic intestinal conditions. These tests are of diagnostic value but are not pathognomonic of grass sickness.

162 (a) Papillomatosis, which is infectious. The causative virus is capable of survival in yards and stables.
(b) Surgical removal of larger warts.
(c) To prevent further corneal damage. There is already a corneal laceration, caudal to the large wart.
(d) Usually these types of papilloma are self-limiting and drop off about 4 months after their first appearance.

163 The horse shows ventral abdominal oedema which may be due to hypoproteinaemia, a local or systemic circulatory disorder or be a sequel to a ventral midline incision. The following should be considered in the differential diagnosis:
● Starvational hypoproteinaemia.
● Malabsorption syndrome.
● Protein-losing conditions, e.g. protein-losing enteropathy.
● Chronic hepatic cirrhosis.
● Local circulatory interference.
● Lymphosarcoma.
● Surgery.
● Congestive heart failure.

164 (a) See *Figure 293*: deep digital flexor tendon (A); medial and lateral branches of the superficial digital flexor tendon (B); straight sesamoidean ligament (C).
(b) There is echodense material subcutaneously. There is an unusual amount of fluid

(echolucent) within the flexor tendon sheath. There is an echodense band crossing the tendon sheath running from the palmar aspect of the deep digital flexor tendon. There is a large hypoechoic lesion in the centre of the palmar aspect of the deep digital flexor tendon.
(c) Synovial fluid analysis of fluid from the tendon sheath to include total and differential white blood cell counts and assessment of cellular morphology, total protein concentration and Gram stain. (The total white blood cell count was 8×10^9/l with 60% polymorphonuclear leucocytes. Total protein concentration was 17 g/l.)
(d) The horse has sustained a penetrating injury of the flexor tendon sheath and the deep digital flexor tendon. The degree of lameness shown by the horse, together with the result of synovial fluid analysis, would tend to mitigate against septic tenosynovitis. The degree of lameness could probably be explained by the original trauma and adhesion formation. None the less, continued systemic antimicrobial therapy is probably warranted, combined with non-steroidal anti-inflammatory drugs, controlled exercise and passive manipulation of the distal limb joints to try to stretch forming adhesions.
(e) Prognosis: guarded to fair; chronic fibrosis is likely which may result in mechanical lameness.

165 (a) The animal has a seedy toe, with evidence of dirt packing between the wall and the sole as a result of the separation at the white line.
(b) A radiograph would show the degree of secondary pedal osteitis present.
(c) If the animal is lame, as a result of infection tracking up the dorsal wall of the hoof, this may cause problems when attempts are made to lever the hoof into a normal position by means of a shoe with a toe extension.

166 (a) Recent work reported that equine muscle glycogen levels may be affected by adjusting diet and training (not just diet alone), i.e feeding a low-carbohydrate diet during exhaustive high-intensity exercise for 5 days to effect glycogen depletion, followed by a high-carbohydrate diet during a 3-day repletion period. However, these findings are controversial, with other workers showing that supplementation of a normal diet, either orally or via an intravenous infusion of glucose, has no effect on glycogen repletion rates following exercise or on the final glycogen concentration reached. In addition, the horse has already very high muscle glycogen concentrations compared to man.
(b) In man it has been suggested that increased muscle glycogen stores may be correlated to increased performance and that glycogen loading may be very beneficial to long-distance athletes, with up to 37% increase in their anaerobic performance. The importance or value of glycogen loading or increased glycogen muscle stores in the horse has not been proven. Several of the papers written on this subject in the horse do not stand up to objective scientific scrutiny and until methods have been developed to assess performance objectively over various race distances (run at times similar to those seen in races), no true evaluation of the importance or otherwise of the various ergogenic aids, such as glycogen loading, can be made.
(c) Glycogen loading could potentially result in laminitis, endotoxaemia, and increased intracellular water retention. Increased glycogen stores, if they truly can be obtained in the horse, could even result in a decreased performance, especially in the sprinter.

167 The 'holding injection' is the name popularly given to human chorionic gonadotrophin (hCG). This is a hormone which is very similar in composition and action to pituitary luteinising hormone (LH). When administered to mares with mature follicles, this preparation is thought to hasten ovulation. However, since the treatment is invariably given at a time when ovulation might normally be expected to occur, a true estimate of its efficacy cannot be made.

The hormone does not increase the mare's chances of conceiving, apart from its possible role in ensuring that ovulation occurs close to the mating day. Recently, analogues of gonadotrophin-releasing hormone have become available and are used for a similar purpose; they are probably less effective than hCG because singly administered doses do not stimulate the pulsatile release that occurs *in vivo*. This drug is also sometimes called the 'holding injection'. Despite the fact that there is no evidence that the 'holding injection' increases the likelihood of the mare conceiving, once such treatment has appeared effective, owners usually request that it be repeated.

168 (a) Pelvic flexure impaction. Sometimes the transverse colon is impacted as well but cannot be palpated.
(b)
- Analgesia. Phenylbutazone is usually effective. (2 g/450 kg intravenously). Xylazine and detomidine are short acting and depress motility. Butorphanol depresses propulsive motility and increases segmental activity so is not indicated for impactions.
- Laxative. Liquid paraffin (4–8 l by stomach tube) may be repeated every 12–24 h. Irritants are too risky in most cases.
- Management. Allow water. Electrolytes can be added. Restrict feed intake or starve. Prevent bedding eating. Beware of dehydration which would necessitate intravenous therapy. Be alert for signs of septic shock which would herald intestinal ischaemia. Be patient.
(c)
- Check teeth.
- Check anthelmintic programme.
- Check feeding and drinking arrangements.
- Does he eat his bed?

169 (a)
- Trim hair from the skin edges. Clean and flush wound with normal saline.
- Tranquillise the horse with, for example, detomidine and butorphanol, and locally infiltrate edges of the wound with a non-irritant local anaesthetic (e.g. 1% mepivacaine without adrenaline).
- Thoroughly clean the wound again and suture skin back into normal apposition with single interrupted non-absorbable sutures; leave a drainage hole at the most distal aspect.
- Place deeper tension sutures over tubing to prevent tension on skin edges.
- Place bandage and dressing on wound and bandage from coronet to above the top of the wound.
- Initiate antimicrobial therapy. Early use of non-steroidal anti-inflammatory drugs (e.g. phenylbutazone) may help to prevent the development of excessive soft-tissue swelling.
(b) Yes. The horse should be kept confined and given antibiotics for 5 days; if possible, the bandages should be left intact for the first 5 days; daily or alternate-day dressing will depend on drainage and exudate.

170 (a) There may be evidence of anaemia but this finding is non-specific. Abnormalities of the clotting cascade are unusual and other diagnostic tests are more likely to reveal the cause of haemorrhage.
(b) Radiographic and endoscopic examinations should be carried out to try to establish the site and cause of bleeding. While it is possible that this sign is due to guttural pouch mycosis or to focal bleeding within the nasal cavity from polyps or neoplasia, it was found to be due to persistent trauma from a chain which struck the horse across the nose during transport. No lesions were found which could otherwise explain the epistaxis, and securing of the chain resulted in a cessation of the epistaxis!

171 The history, clinical and post-mortem features of this case are highly suggestive of non-steroidal anti-inflammatory drug (NSAID) toxicity due to excessive doses of flunixin meglumine administered postoperatively. Although more widespread alimentary tract ulceration and GI loss of plasma proteins is more commonly associated with NSAID toxicity in the horse, a more localised disease (right dorsal colitis) is also occasionally observed. Ulcerative colitis of the right dorsal colon is most likely to occur when horses that are dehydrated are given NSAIDs. Painful musculoskeletal problems are known to interfere with the ability of horses to hydrate adequately. This horse received excessively high doses of flunixin meglumine (recommended dose of flunixin is 1 mg/kg daily; this horse received two to three times this dose).

172 (a) 30° maxillary oblique view with the affected side down.
(b) There is an endotracheal tube in place and the jaws are separated. There is a generalised mineralised opacity (maxillary osteitis) surrounding the area dorsal to the fifth upper cheek tooth and fourth alveolar socket, which is comparatively radiolucent. The fourth upper cheek tooth is absent; however, there is a narrow rectangular radiopacity consistent with dental tissue overlying the caudal part of the fourth alveolar socket just rostral to the fifth cheek tooth and extending almost to the surface of the sky-lined maxillary dental arcades.
(c) A dental sequestrum remains from the incomplete removal of the fourth upper cheek tooth. The presence of this tissue will predispose to orosinus fistulation and continued contamination of the maxillary sinus cavity with ingesta. The secondary sinusitis will therefore persist, resulting in a continued nasal discharge.

173 (a) Respiratory acidosis with good oxygenation.
(b) Treatment consists of intermittent positive pressure ventilation to decrease the arterial carbon dioxide tension. Sodium bicarbonate will only serve to increase the carbon dioxide tension and so will aggravate the situation. Metabolic acidosis would be characterised by a low pH and normal or low $P\text{CO}_2$. Sodium bicarbonate would be the symptomatic treatment of choice in such an instance.

174 (a) Oesophageal choke. Look out for foreign bodies, neurological problems causing dysphagia or, more rarely, acute grass sickness.
(b)
- Antispasmolytic (e.g. hyoscine N-butylbromide and dipyrone) will occasionally be enough to clear the mild case.
- Lavaging the obstruction by stomach tube should be tried but with *great care*. Sedation is helpful. Use liquid paraffin for sugar beet cases, otherwise water. Water can be pumped down a small stomach tube inside a large one. Cuffed nasogastric tubes are a possibility. If in doubt soften ingesta and leave 12 h before repeating.

General anaesthesia can be used as a last resort.
- Antibiotics are a sensible precaution. There is often spillage into the trachea.
- Rehydration intravenously may be necessary in long-standing cases. It gives you time to deal with the oesophagus more gently.

(c)
- Rasp teeth.
- Check feeding regimen.
- Check for other causes, e.g. neurological problems, oesophageal disease. Contrast radiography and endoscopy may be indicated for recurrent cases.

175 (a) The clinical features of this case are typical of chronic eosinophilic gastroenteritis. Diagnosis is confirmed by histological examination of biopsy samples (skin or bowel wall). Most cases do not show eosinophilia of the blood.
(b) The aetiology of the disease is unknown. It is probably a myeloproliferative disorder, showing some similarities to the hypereosinophilic syndromes of man. There is no known effective treatment.

176 Serum protein electrophoresis may be helpful in the identification or *Strongyles vulgaris* larval damage. Protein electrophoresis permits the identification of elevated specific globulin fractions. The beta-1 fraction may be elevated in cases of otherwise inapparent parasitism of this type.

177 (a) The horse shows severe weight loss/cachexia. There is marked hypertrophy of the thoracic expiratory muscles (a 'heave line'). The elbows are abducted, a so-called air hunger sign.
(b) Severe obstructive pulmonary disease, possibly accompanied by emphysema, could account for all the clinical signs. There may also be a concurrent cause of weight loss!
(c) The long-term prognosis is poor in view of the severity of the clinical signs. There may well be both functional and structural alterations of the lungs. Emergency attention to air hygiene, the use of bronchodilators, mucolytics and possibly corticosteroids may bring about a significant improvement.

178 (a) The dyspnoea is probably due to dorsal pharyngeal compression, the most likely cause of which is an enlargement of one or both of the auditory tube diverticula (guttural pouches).
(b) Guttural pouch empyema, guttural pouch tympany.
(c) Radiography and endoscopy of the pharynx and guttural pouches should be performed. In cases of empyema of the guttural pouches an accumulation of fluid will result in a fluid line or lines seen on lateral radiographs. The character and amount of the exudate may be assessed by endoscopy. With tympany of the auditory tube diverticula, one or both of the guttural pouches is overdistended with air. Radiographically, the auditory tube diverticulum extends further caudally than normal, beyond the caudal aspect of the first cervical vertebra. As both guttural pouches may be affected, in many cases all diagnostic methods should be directed towards both.

179 (a) The medial femoral condyle.
(b) Local analgesia of the medial femorotibial joint usually produces an improvement in the animal's gait, and is the most reliable guide. However, a negative response does not preclude a subchondral bone cyst in this location as a cause of lameness. Some animals will exhibit slight distension of the medial femorotibial joint. Other diagnostic

information is highly non-specific for localisation of the pathology. Nuclear scintigraphy is usually negative.

(c) The first technique involves evacuation of the cyst cavity and packing this with an autogenous cancellous bone graft. In the second technique the cyst is again evacuated but the cavity is not packed. It may, however, be supplemented by the creation of portals into the adjacent epiphyseal cancellous bone (forage). The first technique is performed via an arthrotomy and the second either by arthrotomy or arthroscopically.

(d) Radiographic evaluation of the contralateral femorotibial joint, since a significant percentage of cases are bilaterally affected.

180 (a) Either *Tabanid* spp., a large fly, which does not lay eggs on horses legs, or a bot fly, which lays eggs on the jowl, neck, legs and occasionally the abdomen.

(b)
- To destroy the eggs, wash the legs with warm water containing 0.5% malathion or 0.06% coumaphos – use rubber gloves when applying.
- Recommend yearly treatment with anthelmintics, such as ivermectin or trichlorfon, given in the autumn and early winter to kill any larvae in the stomach.

(c) Moisture and warmth from the horse's mouth rubbing the areas where eggs have been laid.

(d) Larvae penetrate the lip, skin or, more usually, the mucosa around the mouth and are eventually swallowed, developing in the stomach before being passed out in the faeces.

181 (a) The trace shows two consecutive P-waves which are not followed by QRS complexes. This is an example of second degree atrioventricular (AV) block. After the two blocked beats the P–P interval shortens and then lengthens prior to the next non-conducted P-wave. This is indicative of sinus arrhythmia. The longest P–Q interval occurs prior to the non-conducted P-wave (Type 1 Wenckebach AV block). The T-wave after the next conducted P-wave following a non-conducted P-wave is smaller than in successive beats. T-wave morphology in the horse is heart rate dependent, and is often different in amplitude after a long pause.

All of these features are indicative of high vagal tone.

(b) This trace may represent transient postexercise sinus arrhythmia which occurs most commonly after a period of light exercise. It would be advisable to re-examine this animal after a period of more sustained work.

(c) This arrhythmia is due to vagal activity associated with heart rate slowing. It is not clinically significant.

182 (a) Abdominal paracentesis. In this case the procedure produced a copious flow of sanguinous fluid with a protein content of 26 g/l and a red blood cell volume of 2%. Paracentesis is extremely helpful to detect whether irreversible tissue damage is taking place.

(b) The condition requires immediate laparotomy. A strangulated herniation of 1.5 m of distal jejunum was found in the epiploic foramen. Obvious ischaemia and devitalisation of bowel required resection and anastomosis.

(c)
- Severe unrelenting pain even in the face of repeated analgesia.
- Rectal findings indicative of a small intestinal obstruction.
- The presence of gastric reflux.
- Absence of intestinal motility.
- Paracentesis producing sanguinous fluid.

(d) The liberal use of flunixin meglumine, a potent inhibitor of prostaglandin synthesis, has masked the horse's clinical response to endotoxaemia in the presence of ischaemic bowel lesions. The apparent stability of the cardiovascular system may result in considerable delay before a surgical decision is taken.

183 (a) Only one mammary gland and teat is present! The skin of the remaining gland and the adjacent area of thigh and ventral abdomen show multiple focal lesions and some swelling.
(b) The lesions are multiple, focal and coalescing nodules and many have ulcerated centres revealing a small amount of purulent material. Histologically, the lesions may be identifiable as necrogranulomata.
(c) The horse probably has generalised granulomatous disease. Other clinical signs include local lymph node enlargement and weight loss, dullness and inappetence.
(d) The condition may be associated with tuberculous infections; therefore direct Ziel–Nielsen-stained smears and culture of material from lesions for possible acid-fast organisms should be performed.

184 (a) The mare's placenta is diffuse, i.e. it occupies the whole of the endometrial surface after 3 months. This is different from the cow in which placental attachment only occurs at the placentomes and the unattached allantochorion between the placentomes can be 'slipped' during uterine palpation. *Figure 294A* shows the ventral surface of a uterus containing a 5-month pregnancy. The outline of the fetus can be seen. Careful incision of the uterus allowed it to be separated from the chorioallantoic membrane (*Figure 294B*). The chorioallantois occupies the whole of the uterine lumen and the diffuse nature of the placenta can be seen. Villi do not develop where the chorioallantois is adjacent to openings of the cervix and fallopian tubes and to the endometrial cups. There were also avillous folds in the chorioallantois which straightened out when the uterus was removed. Incision of the chorioallantois allows the fetus to be seen within the amnion (*Figure 294C*); there is no fusion between this membrane and the allantois.
(b) Fremitus does occur in the uterine artery in later pregnancy but it is not consistent. However, detection of fremitus as an indicator of pregnancy is not necessary in the mare as, unlike in the cow, the uterus remains detectable per rectum throughout gestation. This is because the dorsal surface of the uterus remains dorsal while the uterus enlarges during pregnancy because of the relatively high lateral attachment of the broad ligaments. The ovaries also, therefore, remain dorsal to the uterus and can be palpated into mid-pregnancy, when they are displaced cranially and medially.

185 (a) Infective arthritis or possibly severe trauma. The leucocyte count in the smear prepared when the animal was 2 weeks of age was $51.3 \times 10^9/l$, and 96% of these were neutrophils. This is consistent with infection. It would also be useful to do a Gram stain.
(b) The animal will have received broad-spectrum antibiotics and the joint should also have been flushed one or more times with sterile electrolyte solutions. In this case, the joint was flushed three times over the 2-week period, and the animal was given Timentin for 1 week, followed by penicillin and neomycin for a further 12 days.
(c) The smear made when the animal was 4 weeks of age shows predominantly mononuclear cells and, therefore, the problem has been controlled. The leucocyte count was $1.5 \times 10^9/l$, and 87% of these were mononuclear cells at this stage.

186 (a) The major finding is a markedly raised serum glutamate dehydrogenase (GLDH) level, which is a specific indicator of hepatocellular damage. Aspartate aminotransferase (AST) is only slightly raised but is not a very sensitive indicator of equine hepatic disease. Low blood urea is also consistent with hepatic failure and is due to lack of urea production from ammonia. Hypoalbuminaemia with hyperglobulinaemia (especially beta globulins) is common in hepatic disease but is not pathognomonic. Bilirubin may sometimes be close to normal in equine liver failure and this finding is compatible with the high GLDH level. Overall the findings indicate significant hepatic damage.

(b) Additional investigation would include demonstration of impaired liver function by serum bile acid assay and/or a Bromsulphthalein (BSP) dye clearance test. If evidence of impaired function is obtained, a liver biopsy is indicated.

187 (a) The examiner has torn the full thickness of the bowel wall (*Figure 295*).

(b) Rectal tears occur most often in the dorsal aspect of the rectum, between the 10 and 12 o'clock positions. The direction is usually longitudinal. Most tears are near the pelvic inlet, a distance of 25–30 cm from the anus, which means that they communicate with the peritoneal cavity.

(c)
- The horse should be well tranquillised with detomidine (Domosedan, 0.02–0.03 mg/kg intravenously) and butorphanol (Torbugesic, 0.1 mg/kg intravenously).
- The use of hyoscine-*N*-butylbromide and dipyrone (Buscopan compositum, 0.05 ml/kg intravenously) or propantheline bromide (Proban B, 0.07 mg/kg intravenously) assists in further relaxation of the rectum to facilitate faecal evacuation. Alternatively, epidural anaesthesia (5–10 ml of 2% lidocaine) or a lidocaine enema (10 ml in 50 ml saline) can be used. Epidural anaesthesia adds the benefits of anal relaxation but can cause temporary ataxia.
- 2–4 mg of atropine intravenously will abolish peristalsis and minimise the risk of faecal contamination.
- Careful rectal palpation is performed with the bare hand to enable a more accurate assessment of the internal damage.
- The area of the tear can be packed temporarily with an antiseptic-soaked gauze pack.

(d) The three most important factors are:
- The location of the tear.
- The size of the lesion.
- The number of tissue layers penetrated.

The tear is classified according to the layers torn:
- Grade 1 = mucosa, or mucosa and submucosa.
- Grade 2 = muscularis alone.
- Grade 3 = mucosa, submucosa and muscularis, including tears into the dorsal mesentery and retroperitoneal fossa.
- Grade 4 = complete tear of the rectal wall into the abdominal cavity.

(e)
- The owner must be notified immediately that this is a life-threatening condition with a guarded-to-poor prognosis. An immediate decision regarding therapy or euthanasia should be made.
- High levels of broad-spectrum antibiotics should be administered to all cases. Close monitoring is necessary for early recognition of shock. Fluid therapy must be initiated to counter the effects of endotoxaemia.

- *Grade 1* tears are amenable to medical treatment alone.
- *Grade 2* rectal tears are mainly a theoretical consideration and manageable with dietary control (laxative diet).
- *Grade 3 and 4* tears dictate prompt surgical intervention or immediate euthanasia if gross contamination of the abdominal cavity is present.

Surgical options include:

- Direct suture through laparotomy for ventral tears more than 25 cm cranial to the anus.
- Direct suture through the rectum for tears extending into the dorsal mesentery that are inaccessible via laparotomy. The procedure is facilitated by the use of long-handled needle holders and an expandable rectal speculum. Another method of direct closure through the rectum involves a midline laparotomy to allow an assistant to telescope the bowel over the tip of a rectally inserted Caslick speculum.
- The use of a temporary diverting colostomy allows the terminal small colon and rectum to be kept free of faeces for 2–4 weeks. This leaves the tear to heal spontaneously. A second surgical interference is necessary to re-anastomose the transected colon ends.
- The placement of a temporary indwelling rectal liner. This is anchored to the small colon, proximal to the tear, via a midline laparotomy.

188 Facial palsy. The horse shows flaccidity of the auricular, palpebral, buccal and nasolabial muscles. The fact that all the muscle groups are affected points to a lesion which is either central, i.e. involving the facial nucleus in the medulla oblongata, or which involves the trunk of the nerve before it divides after leaving the skull at the stylomastoid foramen. In the horse illustrated the cause was an osteoma of the styloid process of the hyoid bone. This lesion, which compressed the facial nerve, could be seen by endoscopy of the auditory tube diverticulum (*Figure 296*).

189 (a)
- Debride all damaged tissue and treat as an open wound, allowing it to heal by second intention.
- Remove as little skin as possible.

(b) Yes. Large defects can occur and some loss of extension can occur but most of these injuries heal without loss of performance ability, although the horse may have a subtle adaptation of gait.

(c) The wound could take up to 4 months to repair fully. The horse should be given controlled graded exercise and should be confined to a stall as little as possible. However, uncontrolled turn out in a large area is undesirable. The ideal solution is confinement to a pen or large yard combined with daily walking.

190 (a) Lactation during pregnancy usually indicates placental separation. Most commonly this is caused by the death of one of twins, but may sometimes be the result of bacterial or mycotic placentitis, which starts at the cervical end of the uterus and progresses cranially. The result is almost always abortion. Viral abortion caused by equine herpesvirus 4 is usually rapid, with no premonitory signs, and often a live fetus is expelled; it is wise but sometimes economically impossible to check for the aetiology after any abortion.

(b) Haemorrhage through the vulva is often interpreted by mare owners as a sign of impending abortion, presumably because this is often the case in the human. However, the equine placenta is epitheliochorial, and separation does not cause haemorrhage, so that this sign is not associated with 'threatened abortion' and should not be diagnosed as such.

Invariably, vulval haemorrhage during pregnancy is associated with varicosities and rupture of veins in the region of the hymen (these are occasionally also seen in non-pregnant mares). During pregnancy there is no treatment; haemorrhage is inconsequential in volume although the owner often sees large amounts expelled, especially in the morning (after accumulation during an inactive night). Following parturition the lesions resolve (in non-pregnant mares these vessels may require ligation or cautery).

191 (a) NO! It is most likely to be a thyroid adenoma; most of these are non-functional and are merely unsightly. Estimation of thyroid hormones and stimulation tests are generally normal.
(b) Few other lesions occur here. Local abscessation of pharyngeal lymph nodes may occur in *Streptococcus equi* infection (strangles).
(c) Swelling outside the larynx would not normally cause any interference with air flow through the pharynx or upper airway. Growth is generally slow and can easily be accommodated by the soft tissues laterally! In this case the other gland was normal.

192 (a) In the normal horse, the plasma glucose is expected to rise to reach a maximum level at 120 min, which is approximately double the resting concentration, and then decline again to return to the resting level by 6 h.
(b) The results are consistent with a state of small intestinal malabsorption. There is no appreciable increase in the plasma glucose concentration after administration of the glucose solution.
(c) The diseases which most commonly result in small intestinal malabsorption in adult horses include granulomatous enteritis, chronic eosinophilic gastroenteritis, alimentary lymphosarcoma and villous atrophy.
(d) The prognosis for most cases of small intestinal malabsorption is very poor. A 'flat' absorption response, such as is seen in this example, is generally associated with a severe infiltrative lesion of the intestinal mucosa (e.g. granulomatous enteritis or alimentary lymphosarcoma).

193 (a) Differential diagnoses of mandibular swelling: eruption pseudocysts, submandibular lymph node enlargement and abscessation, periapical dental abscessation, fractured jaw, mandibular bone cyst, neoplasia.
(b)
• Ventral cortical mandibular swelling.
• Loss of periodontal membrane around the rostral dental radical.
• Clubbing of the rostral dental radical.
• Radiolucent halo around the rostral dental radical.
Diagnosis – periapical abscessation of rostral root of third mandibular cheek tooth and associated sinus tract.

194 (a) Uveal cyst.
(b) Iris melanoma.
(c) None.

195 (a) Caudocranial and lateromedial views.

(b) The proximal aspects of the trochlear ridges of the femur have an irregular outline, but the underlying bone is of regular opacity. The trochlear ridges are of similar size (whereas in the adult the medial trochlear ridge is larger). The patella also has an irregular outline. This radiographic appearance is typical of incomplete ossification; ossification of the trochlear ridges of the femur is not complete until 3–5 months of age. Infection can result in a similar radiographic appearance in the early stages but may also result in destruction of subchondral bone.

(c) Intra-articular infection, trauma, osteochondrosis, other.

(d)

- Measure rectal temperature; perform a comprehensive clinical examination with special reference to the umbilicus and the thorax and all other joints.
- Collect synovial fluid from the femoropatellar joint and measure total protein concentration, total and differential white blood cell counts and red cell count. Perform a Gram stain and attempt bacterial culture.
- Perform routine haematology (total and differential white blood cell counts, total protein and albumin concentrations) and measure fibrinogen and IgG.

(e) The patella is fully ossified by 4 months of age; the distal femoral physis closes by 24–30 months of age.

196 (a) Measure the complete blood count (CBC) and plasma fibrinogen. Aspirate the joint aseptically and perform cytology and culture on the fluid obtained. Perform blood cultures. Radiograph the joint for future comparison. Carefully examine the limbs for other foci of infection and the lungs for a pneumonic process. Perform an ultrasonographic examination of the umbilicus.

(b) Septic arthritis with or without osteomyelitis.

(c) Broad-spectrum antibiotics should be administered while awaiting culture results. The umbilicus may be managed medically, by cauterisation using silver nitrate sticks. Possibly, consider local joint therapy (aspirate and flush the joint with a balanced polyanionic electrolyte solution).

197 (a)

- Lice infestation – most likely *Damalinia equi* (small lice) or the more easily seen *Haematopinus asini*.
- Chorioptic mites.
- Harvest mites or chigger mites, scrub itch mites.
- Poultry red mites (proximity to, or being housed, in poultry shed).

(b)

- Whole-body spray, 5–10 l per horse.
- Repeat in 14–16 days.
- Use sprays in accordance with each manufacturer's direction:
  0.45% coumaphos; 0.04% diazinon; 0.62% maldison; 0.1% chlorfenvinphos; all are toxic chemicals and must be used with caution.

198 (a) The lesion is restricted to the area of the parotid salivary gland and is well circumscribed. Lesions of this type seldom cause a cough but the presence of epistaxis is of concern. The origin of the bleeding would need to be established but it is unlikely that the two are related.

(b) The most likely diagnosis is a parotid or auditory tube diverticulum (ATD) (guttural pouch) melanoma/melanosarcoma, which are generally restricted to grey horses.

(c) Melanomas may be relatively benign and slow growing but may be widely disseminated; the presence of other lesions may be significant. Melanomas are frequently found in the perineum and may be of little significance in this site. However, lesions arising in the parotid area may do so from primary lesions in the ATDs (guttural pouches) or from primary melanosarcoma in the parotid salivary glands and may be highly malignant. The prognosis for the horse is extremely guarded.

199 (a) The serosal haemorrhages arise from penetration into the intestinal wall of third-stage, large strongyle larvae. Such lesions may arise in either the small or large intestine and they are generally attributed to infection by *Strongylus vulgaris*. Most texts describe a similar entity of a diffuse, serosal, haemorrhagic reaction specifically sited in the wall of the ileum, known as *Haemolasma ilei*, which is usually attributed to *Strongylus edentatus* infection. In the mucosa and submucosa adjacent to these haemorrhagic serosal lesions there is a severe inflammatory cell reaction and widespread thrombosis of small arteries.
(b) Strongyle infections in general, and intestinal infarction due to *S. vulgaris* in particular, have been associated with colic in the horse.
 In young foals an acute syndrome of pyrexia, anorexia, dullness and colic may occur with recently acquired heavy infection of large strongyle larvae.
 In older animals weight loss, pyrexia and colic are usually associated with slightly later stages of larval migration, classically with arteritis of the cranial mesenteric artery due to the presence of fourth-stage *S. vulgaris* larvae. In these cases the colic may be intermittent or recurrent and there may be an attendant peritonitis. The traditional view that the mesenteric arteritis gives rise to thromboemboli which occlude intestinal arteries has recently been refuted. It now seems more likely that the intestinal ischaemia is a result of diffuse vasoconstriction or intravascular coagulation at the level of the bowel wall and that this may reflect either hypersensitivity or neurohumoral responses to the parasites.

200 (a) Unilateral transverse rostral ramus fracture of the mandible at the level of the diastema with possible involvement of the developing tooth head of the right lateral incisor; ventral and left displacement of incisor arcade.
(b) Anorexia, mandibular swelling, instability and left lateral displacement of mandibular incisor arcade with malocclusion, and compound fracture lacerating the oral mucosa.
(c) Interdental wiring. Following lavage of the oral wound using dilute povidone–iodine solution and removing any bony fragments, the fracture is reduced, ensuring correct dental occlusion and a normal incisor bite. Stainless steel wire (18 gauge) is weaved between the incisors through the interdental spaces at the base of the teeth. The fracture is stabilised using the tension band principle. The wire is fixed immediately rostral to the first mandibular cheek teeth. The sharpened ends of the wire are turned down to prevent laceration of the tongue. A bilateral mental nerve block may supplement postoperative analgesia using non-steroidal anti-inflammatory agents. Postoperative management includes systemic antibiotics and daily lavage of the oral laceration. The interdental wire may be removed under sedation, 6–8 weeks postoperatively and after there has been radiographic and clinical evidence of bone union.

201 There are none. Cystic ovaries do not occur in the mare (see question **14**). Mares are sometimes said to be frequently in oestrus and bad tempered at the same time. This is a contradiction in terms; usually the mare is showing some signs which are misinterpreted as signs of oestrus, i.e. clitoral eversion ('winking' or 'showing') and the frequent passage of small amounts of urine. Ill-behaved or bad-tempered mares are often said to be 'marish'; this term seems to imply that they are unpredictable and may kick when not provoked. If owners believe (and this is often suggested by their veterinary surgeon) that the behavioural problem is related to ovarian function, they will often say that it occurs in a cyclic pattern; however, if detailed daily records are kept these rarely support such an assertion.

In reality, mares in oestrus are usually very tractable; they squat, raise their tails, evert the clitoris, urinate – only rarely do they kick, although they may initially be scared of the stallion.

Mares with behavioural anomalies may have a relationship problem with their owner, particularly if the mare is allowed to be dominant, or may be temperamentally unsuitable for the job for which they are required. Ovariectomy will not effect a cure.

202 (a) Peripheral blindness (dilated pupils).
(b) Signs of vestibular and facial nerve involvement following head trauma are usually associated with haemorrhage into the petrous temporal bone and associated fractures of that bone and/or the basilar bones. Another consequence of such head trauma can be an acute amputation-type lesion of the optic nerves, where they enter the optic canals on the floor of the calvarium. Degrees of unilateral or bilateral, partial or total, peripheral blindness occur and the signs are essentially non-reversible. This makes a major difference to the outlook because compensation for signs of vestibular involvement, namely the head tilt, eye deviation and gait abnormality, occurs to a large extent because of normal visual input.

203 (a) Meconium impaction.
(b) Digital examination of the rectum for hard meconium balls and to establish that the tract is patent.
(c) An enema, analgesics if the pain continues, and possibly mineral oil.

204 (a) Particular attention should be paid to auscultation of the lungs in a case with this history. No ventral lung sounds could be auscultated but somes rales could be heard dorsally. Cardiac sounds could be heard over a much wider area than normal. Percussion of the lungs gave the impression of dullness in the lower lung fields.
(b) This history and clinical picture is typical of pleuritis. In many cases pleural sounds are not auscultated because of fluid build-up. Pleuritis often presents as mild-to-moderate colic. Respiratory rate is not necessarily faster unless there is significant lung involvement. Later in its course laboured but quite slow abdominal breathing may be seen (*Figure 297A*):
   Immediate treatment:
- High levels of antibiotics should be administered as soon as possible (e.g. procaine penicillin and trimethoprim sulphadioxine b.i.d.).
- Phenylbutazone or flunixin meglumine are important as anti-inflammatories and analgesics.
Further diagnostic steps should be taken as soon as possible.
- Tracheal aspirate culture, both aerobic and anaerobic, should be performed as well as a cytological examination and a Gram stain of the sample. This may suggest a change in antibiotics.
- Haematology is not so helpful but usually shows a leucocytosis at first. If there is no

immediate clinical improvement or if there is respiratory embarrassment, move on to the following steps.
- Chest X-ray may establish the presence of fluid (*Figure 297B*).
- Thoracocentesis should be used to drain large quantities of pleural fluid (*Figure 297C*) and may need to be repeated; sometimes massive fibrin deposits (*Figure 297D*) develop, making drainage difficult. Submit the fluid for culture, cytology and protein estimation. Ultrasonography may help to localise fluid pockets.
- General management. Avoid stress. Keep the horse warm and comfortable in a dust-free environment and encourage eating and drinking. Act quickly. There is a high mortality rate once pleural effusion develops.

205 (a) Hyperextension of the distal interphalangeal joints, so-called laxity of the deep digital flexor tendons.
(b) The feet should be trimmed and an attempt made to return them to a normal position by shoeing the animal with heel extensions.

206 (a) Postanaesthetic forelimb lameness. It is impossible to distinguish between myopathy and neuropathy from a photograph, but in view of the apparent lack of distress or sweating, and the animal's apparent readiness to eat, a neuropathy is likely. Postanaesthetic myopathies tend to be very painful and cause distress to the animal. Confirmation could be obtained by laboratory estimation of plasma muscle enzyme concentrations, i.e. creatinine kinase (CK) (peaks within 6 h) and aspartate aminotransferase (AST) (peaks within 24 h). Remember that after anaesthesia of 2 h duration, CK and AST are likely to be elevated relative to normal resting values, even in the absence of clinical signs. Values obtained when a horse is still recumbent may be misleading because of inadequate tissue perfusion.
(b) Rest, nursing and analgesics if the animal is in discomfort. If the animal survives the immediate postanaesthetic period, this condition generally slowly resolves with time with no residual lameness. No specific treatment is available. Attempts must be made at prevention, e.g. by careful positioning during anaesthesia, maintenance of arterial blood pressure, good oxygenation and minimal anaesthesia time.

207 (a) Fracture of the olecranon, radial nerve paralysis.
(b) Mediolateral views of the elbow are obtained with the limb to be examined adjacent to the cassette and the limb protracted. Craniocaudal views are obtained either with the limb bearing weight or lifted. In the former position it may be helpful to angle the X-ray beam proximodistally approximately 10–15°.
(c) There is a displaced, complete, articular, slightly comminuted fracture of the olecranon of the ulna.
(d) A = proximal ulnar epiphysis; B = epiphysis of the medial epicondyle of the humerus.
(e) Internal fixation using either a contoured dynamic compression plate (DCP) or Steinmann pins and tension band wires.
(f) The proximal ulnar physis closes at 24–36 months of age, and the proximal radial physis at 11–24 months of age. If a DCP is used care should be taken not to place screws in the proximal radial physis. Plate removal should be considered following fracture repair to avoid disparate growth between the radius and ulna. If Steinmann pins and tension band wires are used these should be removed following fracture repair to avoid premature closure of the ulnar physis.

208 (a) A very upright dorsal hoof wall on the left forelimb, and a small wound on the lateral aspect of the left metacarpophalangeal (fetlock) joint.
(b) The animal is suffering from flexural deformity of the distal interphalangeal joint on the left forelimb, probably secondary to chronic lameness as a result of the advanced degenerative joint disease present in the fetlock joint.
(c) As a result of the low-level chronic lameness present in the left forelimb, the owner had decided to keep this animal for breeding. However, it was felt that the animal had increasing difficulty in using this limb. When held parallel to the other limb, the dorsal hoof wall was past the vertical, and it tended to stand with this limb in front of the other one to try to compensate for this. The hoof axis was corrected by deep digital flexor tenotomy just above the bulbs of the heel. It was felt that this would produce a more immediate, predictable result than section of the accessory ligament of the deep digital flexor tendon (inferior check ligament) and shoeing with a toe extension, as there was concern that the animal would increasingly favour the limb as attempts were made to lever the foot into a more normal position.

209 (a) The palmar and distal medial and lateral aspects of the limb are finely clipped and washed and ultrasound coupling gel is liberally applied. The body of the suspensory ligament is examined in both transverse and longitudinal planes using a 7.5 MHz transducer (linear or sector scanner), from the palmar aspect of the limb. A stand off is not required. The medial and lateral branches of the suspensory ligament are examined from the palmar medial and palmar lateral aspects of the limb; due to the more superficial location of the suspensory ligament branches a stand off is required.
(b) *Figure 162A* shows that the body of the suspensory ligament, in the region of its division, is diffusely hypoechoic laterally. *Figures 162B–E* shows that the lateral branch of the suspensory ligament is enlarged distally (*Figures D* and *E*) and has an area of reduced echogenicity throughout its length.
(c) Radiographic examination of the metacarpophalangeal joint to assess particularly the lateral proximal sesamoid bone.

   Pain associated with the suspensory ligament is difficult to eliminate fully by perineural analgesia. There is frequently pain caused by passive flexion of the metacarpophalangeal joint in association with suspensory ligament desmitis. In this case there may also be pain associated with the metacarpophalangeal joint *per se* in view of the joint capsule distension. Thus, consideration could be given to assessing the effect of intra-articular analgesia; however, this was not performed at this stage since many normal event horses have distended fetlock joint capsules and low grade pain immediately following an event (see question **226**).

210 (a) Severe diarrhoea in adult horses is a significant clinical sign and may be responsible for the lethargy. The lameness is unlikely to be directly related.
(b) Possible conditions which may be responsible include: parasitism (particularly cyathostomiasis), salmonellosis, equine malabsorption syndrome, granulomatous enteritis, dietary imbalances and liver failure.
(c)
- Faecal examination for parasite eggs and bacteria.
- Rectal biopsy for bacterial culture and histological examination. Test treatments with anthelmintics may be useful as a diagnostic aid.
- D-Xylose (or glucose) absorption tests.
- A full haematological profile should be undertaken. Parasitic conditions may show significant anaemia, hyperproteinaemia (increased beta-2 globulins).

- Malabsorption syndromes and protein-losing enteropathies result in hypoproteinaemia. Cardiorespiratory function might need to be investigated if lethargy is unrelated to diarrhoea.
- A full lameness work-up should be undertaken.

211 (a) Packed cell volume, total plasma protein, icterus index. The foal has yellow mucous membranes and this combined with lethargy, weakness and elevated heart rate is suggestive of haemolytic anaemia.

(b) Neonatal isoerythrolysis (NI) is the most likely. Other possibilities include septicaemia, liver failure, biliary atresia, congenital viral infection (herpes). Tyzzer's disease usually occurs in slightly older foals (7–40 days old).

(c) Packed red blood cell (RBC) transfusion (throughly washed red blood cells from the dam), or whole blood transfusion (from a compatible donor), if the foal is showing signs related to anaemia.

(d) The likelihood of the mare producing another NI foal is high. Screen the mare late in gestation for anti-RBC antibodies; mix colostrum at birth with RBC from the newborn foal (using jaundice foal agglutination test) to detect incompatibility. If the mare is suspected of having antibodies against the foal's RBCs, prevent the foal from nursing the mare's colostrum, and provide an alternative source of colostrum. Attend the delivery, milk out the dam every hour, muzzle the foal for at least 24 h (48 h preferred) and provide donor colostrum within the first 6 h of life.

212 (a) *Onchocerca* infestation.

(b)
- Biopsy as fresh a lesion as possible.
- Mince biopsy material with Tyrodes' solution for 3 h at 37°C; filter through 250 μ sieve and centrifuge at 3000 rev/min for 5 min.

   Examine residual sediment in suspended droplet chamber for larval worms.

(c) Oral dosage with ivermectin; repeat in 2–3 months.

213 (a) Follicular fluid appears black during ultrasonography. Ovulatory follicles are usually between 3.0 and 5.0 cm diameter, although exceptions can occur. Typically, a mature follicle becomes soft before ovulation; this is detectable on ultrasonography because the surface of the follicle in contact with the transducer becomes flattened due to the pressure of contact necessary to obtain a clear image (*Figures 298A, D* and *G*).

   The 'hazy' white echo at the bottom right, and to a lesser extent the bottom left, of the follicle in *Figure 298A* is an artefact caused by gas in an adjacent loop of bowel (not shown).

(b) The non-oestrous uterus has a relatively homogeneous appearance. During oestrus, the endometrium becomes oedematous and the lymphatics between the endometrium and myometrium become distended. This change is presumably caused by oestrogens, and the intensity of the 'oedematous' change increases as oestrus proceeds. Maximal oedema usually occurs 24–48 h before ovulation. Ultrasonographically, oedema causes the uterus to have a mottled or marbled 'dart-board' appearance. There are alternating dark segments and light strips which correspond to the oedematous (lymphatic) centres and more dense endometrial coverings of uterine folds. *Figures 298M–P* show moderate oedema in the cranial uterine body and uterine horn, respectively. More intense oedema in the mid-body is shown in *Figure 298N*.

(c) After ovulation the recently emptied follicle fills with blood. Static blood (CH) is highly echogenic because the cellular elements overlap and are reflective. This causes an intense white image after 12–24 h (*Figure 298B*). Sometimes the CH has a dark centre due to residual follicular fluid or serum (*Figure 298 E and H*). Over the next few days the 'whiteness' of the CH becomes less intense, and further black areas may develop in its centre, possibly due to serum having been extruded from the thrombus.

(d) By 10 days of age the corpus luteum produces a dull-grey image (*Figure 298C*) and may still contain a black (fluid) central lacuna (*Figure 298F and I*). It is usually highlighted by the presence of small follicles around its periphery.

(e) Occasionally, follicles luteinise without ovulating. An apparently normal follicle may, towards the end of oestrus, become filled with white flecks which represent intra-follicular haemorrhage (*Figure 298J*). The 'follicle' then increases in size, coincident with a more intense swirling 'snowstorm' appearance which soon organises into a static lattice-like appearance within the follicle (*Figure 298K*). The wall of the follicle thickens due to luteinisation of the thecal cells. This phenomenon occurs sporadically in any one mare and at that oestrus she will obviously not conceive as the ovum has not been released. However, the luteal structure thus formed acts like a normal CL and usually is lysed after 14 days. *Figure 298L* shows the luteinised follicle seen in *Figure 298K* 10 days later; the whole structure is considerably smaller and more dense.

(f) Not uncommonly the cyclic CL fails to regress at 14 days. In this case progesterone continues to influence the tubular tract so the uterus becomes tonic, as in early pregnancy, and the cervix remains closed. However, as this condition of prolonged dioestrus proceeds, follicular development becomes more marked as in early pregnancy. These follicles do not influence the tubular tract so that typically many follicles of up to 2.5 cm (one or two may be larger) are imaged and the tubular tract has the homogeneous appearance of progesterone domination. *Figure 298Q and R* are ultrasonograms of the left and right ovaries of a mare in prolonged dioestrus; there are many follicles, and a mature CL in the centre of the right ovary.

214 (a) Gastric tympany from fermentation of grass cuttings. The stomach may be impacted with the grass cuttings.

(b)

- Decompression as often as necessary is crucial. It may be difficult to relieve pressure when the ingesta is frothy. Use a large stomach tube with a fenestrated end. Gastric tympany from any cause is usually very painful. Surgical relief may be necessary but is technically difficult.
- Analgesia. Profound analgesia and sedation will be needed. Xylazine or detomidine work best.
- Laxatives by stomach tube can worsen the gastric distension and should not be used. Agents reducing surface tension, or oral antibiotics, e.g. neomycin, sometimes help.

215 (a) Collapse of either the central or the third tarsal bone dorsally resulting in dorsal displacement of the proximal calcaneus and the curby hock appearance. In this case, the collapse was of the central tarsal bone.

(b) The animal has developed a flexural deformity of the metatarsophalangeal joint, probably as a result of the chronic lameness on this limb.

(c) The owner was advised to confine the mare and foal to a small paddock to help the lameness on this limb to settle down, and to introduce a regimen of controlled walking exercise for the foal once the lameness had improved. The prognosis for athletic function is guarded.

216 (a) Cysts of *Echinococcus granulosus* (equine strain).
(b) The definitive hosts are domestic and wild Canidae. Gravid segments are passed in their faeces. Equines ingest the onchospheres, which penetrate the gut and migrate either in the blood to the liver or in the lymph to the lungs, where they form cysts. The inner germinal layer buds off brood capsules containing scolices. The cycle is completed by ingestion of equine viscera by the definitive host, usually hounds fed equine offal.
(c) An ante-mortem definitive diagnosis could have been made by hepatic ultrasonography, if their presence had been suspected.

217 (a) Palpebral oedema and swelling of the supraorbital fossae are obvious.
(b) Equine viral arteritis and African horse sickness. Abortion is common in both diseases.
(c) Equine viral arteritis is more likely. Additional signs which may be seen in groups of horses include photophobia, lacrimation, corneal oedema, colic and lymphadenopathy. The diseases are difficult to differentiate clinically but fortunately are separated geographically. Serological and virus isolation procedures may be required to confirm either diagnosis. Equine viral arteritis and African horse sickness also present with milder forms which closely resemble the upper respiratory tract virus infections.

218 (a) Aortoiliac thrombosis. The horse is sweating profusely over the cranial part of the body yet the hindquarters are not sweating.
(b) Both murmurs are probably functional in origin and are likely to be of no significance. The localised early systolic murmur over the heart base is likely to be an ejection murmur caused by the rapid flow of blood into the aorta. The early diastolic murmur is probably caused by the rapid flow of blood into the ventricle during filling. Both murmurs are heard commonly in clinically normal horses, especially Thoroughbreds.
(c) Investigation of the saphenous veins immediately after exercise may give an indication of the severity of the condition. Rectal examination of the terminal aorta and iliac arteries may enable palpation of the thrombosis. Palpation of the internal iliac arteries will reveal the presence or absence of a pulse or the presence of fremitus. Ultrasonography of the terminal aorta and iliacs will reveal the extent of the thrombus and the degree of vessel occlusion.
(d) The prognosis is very poor. This degree of incoordination and distress after minimal exercise and the lack of sweating over the hindquarters implies bilateral involvement of the iliac arteries. Anticoagulant therapy is unlikely to be successful in this case. Ultrasonography would confirm the extent of the thrombus and give a more accurate indication of the possible outcome.

219 (a) Only 5–10% of cases have obstructions that require surgery.
(b) Although success rates for colic surgery vary from clinic to clinic, overall survival rates are in the region of 50–60%.
(c) Irreversible bowel ischaemia and endotoxaemia occur within 8 h of small intestinal and 4 h of large intestinal strangulation.
(d) The highest mortality rate exists for 360° torsion of the large colon (69%), followed by epiploic foramen incarceration (57%), ileal impaction (9%) and non-strangulating large colon displacements (7%).

(e) Delay is still the most common cause of failure.
(f) Horses with a heart rate > 100 beats/min in combination with a PCV > 60% rarely survive surgery.

220 (a) Infestation with *Habronema* larvae.
(b)
- Bacterial infections: (i) *Pseudomonas*; (ii) *Klebsiella*.
- Tumour – squamous cell carcinoma.

Scrapings from the urethral process should be examined for the presence of *Habronema* larvae. Often other lesions may be present around the eyes of the same or other horses.
(c) Debride initially, and dress with 50% invermectin + 50% DMSO; drench horse with full dose of ivermectin.
(d) Fertility can be markedly reduced if blood and semen are deposited within the mare's uterus at service.

221 (a) The plasma glucose peaks at 120 min, but the maximum level is significantly lower than double the resting level. This might be described as a 'partial malabsorption' result. It could indicate low grade or focal disease of the small bowel, or might reflect the involvement of extra-intestinal factors (e.g. endocrine factors).
(b) Multiple bowel wall biopsies are indicated to confirm the presence of small intestinal disease.

222 (a) Squamous cell carcinoma/squamous papilloma.
(b) Penile amputation and urethrostomy.
(c)
- Intra- and postoperative haemorrhage from the penile stump or urethrostomy incision; intermittent urethral haemorrhage can be expected for up to 4 weeks postoperatively.
- Postoperative penile and preputial swelling as a result of inadequate haemostasis and haematoma formation or oedema from poor tissue handling and pre-existing balanoposthitis. This will predispose to urethrostomy failure, anuria and possible bladder rupture.
- Incisional infection.
- Urethral extension of the neoplasm.
- Metastatic lymph node involvement.

(d) Biopsy of amputated section, to determine neoplastic nature of lesion, i.e. carcinoma, papilloma or papilloma with premalignant changes, and to evaluate the involvement of the urethral diverticulum and urethra.
- Inguinal lymph node biopsy – reactive hyperplasia or metastatic involvement.
- Presence of pre-existing preputial neoplasia.

(e)
- Local excision.
- Reefing operation.
- Preputial ablation and urethrostomy.
- *En bloc* resection and penile retroversion.

223 (a) Salivation with blood and froth, haemorrhagic nasal discharge, flaring of nostrils.
(b) Difficulty with swallowing or mastication resulting in excessive salivation, foul

smell from the nose associated with the nasal discharge, and dyspnoea as evidenced by the flared nostrils.

(c) It is likely that a haemorrhagic focus associated with a space-occupying lesion is present. Dysphagia may be due to a space-occupying lesion, resulting in pharyngeal obstruction, or due to neurological dysfunction.

(d)
- A careful neurological examination for evidence of cranial nerve dysfunction.
- Endoscopic examination of the upper respiratory tract including the auditory tube diverticula.
- Radiographic examination of the head.

An extensive ethmoid haematoma was identified, which resulted in pharyngeal obstruction and hence dysphagia. There was compromise of the upper airway resulting in dyspnoea.

224 (a) Equine periodic ophthalmia (recurrent uveitis).

(b) History of sudden onset together with clinical signs of photophobia, dull dark iris, constricted pupil and lowered intraocular pressure.

(c) Mydriatics and corticosteroids.

225 (a) Liver fluke – *Fasciola hepatica*. It is relatively unusual to find evidence of liver fluke infection in equine livers in the UK, and experimental studies have shown that the horse is relatively resistant to fluke compared with ruminant species. Generally, donkeys are considered to be more susceptible to liver fluke infection than horses and ponies.

(b) Clinical equine fascioliasis is very uncommon. Infected animals are either asymptomatic or present with vague symptoms such as illthrift, loss of body condition and/or poor athletic performance.

(c)
- Demonstration of fluke eggs in faeces is confirmatory of fascioliasis, but 'false-negative' results may arise if only immature flukes are present or if egg excretion is intermittent, i.e. repeated sampling may be necessary.
- Blood biochemical evidence of a hepatopathy may be detected in fluke-infected animals. Raised plasma levels of liver enzymes such as aspartate transaminase and sorbitol dehydrogenase may arise as a result of migration of immature fluke in hepatic parenchyma, whereas alkaline phosphatase and gamma glutamyl transferase, which indicate biliary tract damage, would be increased if adult fluke were present.
- Adult fluke are haematophagic such that infected animals may have an anaemia.

(d) Triclabendazole – suggested dose rate 15 mg/kg by mouth or stomach intubation. (Note: no flukicidal drugs have UK product licence for use in horses.)

226 (a) There is modelling of the palmar aspect of the lateral proximal sesamoid bone and prominent, broad, radiating lucent lines in the proximal one-half. There is an irregular contour of the dorsomedial proximal aspect of the proximal phalanx.

(b) So-called sesamoiditis – clearly of longer standing than the lameness. Possible degenerative joint disease.

(c) Intra-articular analgesia of the metacarpophalangeal joint. This was performed after box rest for 4 weeks, and reduction of the acute inflammation associated with the suspensory desmitis. Mild lameness persisted which was alleviated by intra-articular analgesia. Intra-articular analgesia is unlikely to remove pain associated with the proximal sesamoid bones *per se*. This supports a diagnosis of concurrent degenerative disease.

(d) The productive bony changes are enthesophytes, caused by chronic tearing of the attachment of the suspensory ligament. The lucent zones adjacent to the vascular channels, but outside the normal bone, are areas of fibrous tissue around nutrient vessels. The condition is an enthesopathy rather than a strictly inflammatory condition of the sesamoid bones.

227 (a) The laceration should be repaired. Removal would expose the lower portion of the eye to further irritation and injury.

(b) The wound could either be repaired with the horse sedated using, for example, detomidine and butorphanol, or xylazine and pethidine, combined with infiltration of the skin edges with a non-irritant local anaesthetic (e.g. mepivacaine 1%, without adrenaline) or with the horse under general anaesthesia. If done standing, it might be useful to perform an auriculopalpebral nerve block, to relax the orbicularis oculi muscles; a supraorbital block will provide analgesia and negate the use of local infiltration of local anaesthetic.

(c)

- 2/0 or 3/0 absorbable material, polygalactin 90 (Vicryl) or polyglycolic acid (Dexon). Use a simple, continuous suture with buried knots.
- Use a simple interrupted pattern with a non-absorbable suture such as polypropylene (Surgilene or Prolene), polygluconate (Raxlon), polydioxanone (PDS) or monofilament polybutyl ester (Novafil).

228 (a) There is marked enlargement at the frontomaxillary suture. Sometimes there is a history of head trauma, but frequently there is not. The horse usually presents with facial swelling; this usually reduces in size but a permanent swelling may persist.

(b) The eyes should be examined carefully. The application of fluoroscein dye might identify the presence of a corneal ulcer or conjunctivitis or suggest obstruction of the nasolacrimal duct. In normal horses the dye may be expected to appear at the nasal opening of the duct after 5–15 min.

(c) The nasolacrimal duct, enclosed in its bony canal, passes close to the inflamed sutures. Local swelling may cause narrowing or deviation of the duct sufficient to result in partial or complete obstruction. Retrograde flushing of the duct may confirm such an obstruction.

229 The mare may not be showing spontaneous signs of oestrus for all the reasons listed in the answer to question **259**. However, at this time of year it is very unlikely that she is still in winter anoestrus or the transition to cyclic activity; immaturity is also not a problem. Apparent failure of treatment may therefore be because:

- The dose of prostaglandin was too small to cause luteolysis; this is unlikely because the recommended doses of commercially available products are usually much greater than those actually required to cause luteolysis in the mare.
- The mare may have a granulosa cell tumour – prostaglandin would not affect the situation.
- A mare in prolonged dioestrus may, at the time of prostaglandin administration and despite the presence of a dominant corpus luteum (CL), have many follicles, some of which could be mature (>3.5 cm diameter). After luteolysis such follicles may regress and be replaced by others which eventually ovulate, or may themselves rupture so soon (within 48 h) that the mare has little chance of showing signs of oestrus. Neither palpation nor ultrasound examination can predict the fate of such follicles. *Figure 299* shows the progesterone concentrations of a mare in prolonged dioestrus;

prostaglandin (PG) caused luteolysis which was followed by ovulation (O) and a luteal phase of normal length.

- If a mare in prolonged dioestrus has a secondary CL less than 5 days old, this will not lyse although the primary CL will.
- If a mare is 'shy' or if the teasing technique is inadequate (often it is a combination of the two), then in physiological oestrus she may not be induced to show clinical signs; she is then said to have 'silent heats'. Many of these mares will 'show' if teased properly and if clinical examination reveals that they are in oestrus the stud will usually spend more time trying to get her mated. 'Silent heats' can occur after effective prostaglandin administration, or may, as in this case, have occurred during June so that prostaglandin may not have been given at an appropriate stage of the cycle; the CL is not responsive to PG during the first 5 days after ovulation.

230 (a) Varus deformity of the carpus, as a result of instability created by fracture of the proximal aspect of the fourth metacarpal bone and subluxation of the second carpal bone.
(b) Stabilisation of the second carpal bone, and reduction and stabilisation of the fourth metacarpal bone fracture.
(c) Prognosis for athletic function is guarded.

231 (a) Tapeworms – *Anoplocephala perfoliata* – which have a predilection for the ileocaecal valve, but they may also be found in the small intestine. The other equine tapeworm *A. magna* occurs less commonly and infects the small intestine.
(b) There have been few detailed studies on the pathogenesis of equine tapeworm infections. Large burdens may be present without causing clinical effects, although erosive or ulcerative mucosal lesions of the distal small intestine or ileocaecal valve are often present. There have been clinical reports associating tapeworm infection with conditions such as caecal perforation/rupture, ileal or caecal intussusception and also ileal hypertrophy.
(c) Definitive diagnosis is made by demonstration of tapeworm eggs in faeces, by use of flotation or sedimentation techniques. Eggs may only be passed intermittently such that examination of several samples collected on consecutive days may be necessary to confirm the diagnosis. Pyrantel embonate at a dose rate of 38 mg/kg (twice the strongyle dose) will effectively remove tapeworm burdens from most horses.

232 Cryptorchid status can be confirmed by the measurement of oestrone sulphate in plasma or by using the human chorionic gonadtrophin (hCG) stimulation test.
Although the oestrone sulphate level can differentiate between cryptorchid horses and those with male-like behaviour that have been effectively castrated (false rigs), this measurement is not suitable for use in horses of less than 3 years, or in donkeys.
Testosterone measurement alone can give equivocal results necessitating further testing. The dynamic test/hCG stimulation test, in which testosterone levels are measured before and after intravenous administration of 6000 iu hCG, may be more useful in identifying unilateral cryptorchids than bilateral cryptorchids.

233 (a) Endogenous losses of sodium have been given as 15–20 mg/kg bodyweight/day in a non-sweating horse. The availability of Na from feedstuffs has been reported as being between 45% and 90%. Therefore requirements for a mature 500-kg non-exercising horse can be calculated as being between 8 g and 22 g of dietary Na per day.

A sodium concentration of at least 0.1% in the maintenance diet has been suggested.
(b) Endogenous losses of Ca have been given as being around 20–25 mg/kg bodyweight/day with a net availability from feedstuffs of between 45% and 70% (except where significant oxalates are present). Therefore requirements for a mature 500-kg non-exercising horse can be calculated as being between 14 g and 28 g of Ca (usually given as between 20 g and 25 g Ca with 15 g P – as the Ca:P ratio is believed to be important as well as the absolute amounts of Ca and P). These values are approximate, as individual variability in absorptive capacity may occur and complex mineral interactions within the gastrointestinal tract may also affect absorption.
(c) Sweat contains low concentrations of Ca (and P) but is hypertonic to plasma with respect to Na (and P and Cl^-), i.e. around 145–160 mmol/l or 3.3–3.7 g/l for Na.
(d) This depends on the environmental conditions, nature of the work, the animal's fitness and to some extent the animal's temperament. In favourable climatic conditions sweat loss can be in the order of 7–8 l/h in long-distance rides. In hot humid conditions, where sweating is partially ineffective, production can be as high as 10–15 l/h. Therefore a fit racehorse tends to loose between 1–5 l in a race and an endurance horse between 25–30 l or more.
(e) For a sweating horse (= 500 kg) doing moderate work (sweat loss = 10 l) the required Na intake based on the above figures would vary from 45 to 104 g/day. Very few horses would be fed or eat 104 g (= 9.5 oz) of salt! (The contents of the gastrointestinal tract may provide an important reservoir for Na during hard work and the electrolyte losses that occur with heavy sweating cannot be restored all at once.) Guidelines tend to be more general and assume the higher level of availability; so for light work around 30 g and for moderate work around 50 g have been recommended (i.e. on hay and compound feed up to around an additional 28 g of NaCl may be required by a horse in moderate work, whereas on an oat/hay diet up to around 100 g additional NaCl may be required).
(f) Requirements for Ca in the exercising horse are even more controversial and confusing, especially if the horse is still growing. Some workers have suggested that any increase with exercise will be met by the obligatory increase in calcium intake due to the increase in dry matter intake. However, others suggest that higher dietary levels of Ca need to be provided for the performance horse. Commonly, recommendations for a mature exercising horse are that it receives approximately twice the amount of Ca than P: around 30–50 g Ca and 15–20 g P. For the young, growing, exercising horse most suggest that far higher levels of Ca are beneficial; however others state they are harmful. The above requirements are approximate and are based on limited and often contradictory work.

234 Don't buy it. The illustration shows two abnormalities: first, entrapment of the epiglottis by the glossoepiglottic mucosa, and second, a major defect of the soft palate. The palatal hypoplasia extends to the right pharyngeal wall (left in *Figure 180*) and therefore it cannot be iatrogenic. Also, out of view, the cartilage flap at the opening of the auditory tube diverticulum was deformed: this is a common finding with congenital palatal defects. To compound matters the motility of the left arytenoid cartilage was highly suspect but this cannot be appreciated from a photograph.
   Although correction of the epiglottal entrapment is straightforward, palatal defects should be regarded as irreparable.

235 (a) The wear pattern on the incisor teeth indicate that the horse is a 'crib biter'.
(b) These horses are often but not always wind suckers (repeated swallowing of air).

(c) It is suggested that acute colic and chronic weight loss are common effects of these vices, although there is little scientific evidence to support this. There may be marked development of the muscles of the ventral neck but this is not likely to result in any pathological signs.

(d) Some horses can be controlled by application of a cribbing strap around the neck just caudal to the jaw. Surgical treatment by cutting the 'strap' muscles of the neck (sternothyrohyoideus, omohyoideus and possibly sternocephalicus) with or without sectioning the ventral branch of the spinal accessory nerve is successful in some horses.

Crib biting is thought to be a stereotypic behaviour and has been controlled by the administration of narcotic antagonists (e.g. naloxane), but this is a palliative rather than curative treatment.

236 (a) 'Sweet itch', *Culicoides* hypersensitivity.
(b)
- *Microsporum gypseum* infection (not pruritic) – culture hairs.
- Psoroptic mange – rarely shows papules: is very itchy and horse will rub tail hairs; find mites in ears, tail and mane.
- Oxyuris infestation – find eggs under tail; responds to anthelmintics.
- *Stomoxys* bites – get papules; rarely rub for more than 24 h; presence of flies.
- *Dermatophilus* – culture; hair plucks out with characteristic appearance.

237 (a) The lucent circle around the metallic opacity in the flexor view of the navicular bone suggests that the lesion has been present for at least 2 weeks. In this case, the injury occurred 25 days before these radiographs were obtained.
(b) The mare has had a penetrating wound to the foot, and a metallic foreign body is present adjacent to the distal horizontal border of the navicular bone.
(c) Euthanasia.

238 (a) The tracheal wash sample shows an intense eosinophilic reaction. This is most commonly observed in cases of lungworm (*Dictyocaulus arnfieldi*) infestation. Infection with this parasite generally occurs when grazing pasture which has also been grazed by donkeys. Asymptomatic patent infections with *D. arnfieldi* occur in a large proportion of donkeys.

D. arnfieldi infections in horses are usually non-patent, and diagnosis is generally not possible by examination of faeces for the parasite larvae. Confirmation of the diagnosis may be achieved by endoscopic examination of the lower airways, when larvae may be observed grossly. Alternatively, larvae may be found in the tracheal wash or bronchoalveolar lavage samples. Response to specific treatment is also a useful aid to diagnosis.
(b) Effective treatment can usually be achieved by a routine dose of ivermectin (200 µg/kg). Affected animals may show a temporary worsening of the clinical signs for 1–2 days before a rapid improvement.

239 (a) Ventricular tachycardia. There is a fast rate, no P-waves, wide and abnormal QRS complexes.
(b) Prognosis must be guarded as this type of rhythm often converts into ventricular fibrillation.
(c) Treatment consists of correction of predisposing factors, e.g. drug overdose, acidosis, hypoxia, by stopping the administration of anaesthetic agent, institution of

intermittent positive pressure ventilation with oxygen-enriched gases and administration of fluids. Lignocaine hydrochloride (without adrenaline) is the drug treatment of choice; 2–4 mg/kg is administered by slow intravenous injection. An infusion of lignocaine (0.02 mg/kg/n.in) may be used to maintain sinus rhythm.

240 (a) This is a transverse ultrasonogram of the palmar metacarpal soft tissues obtained using a stand off. In the left-hand picture there appears to be an hypoechoic region in the accessory ligament of the deep digital flexor tendon (inferior check ligament), but this may be an artefact and should be re-evaluated without a stand off. (It was not detectable.) In the right-hand picture there is an echolucent rim palmar to the superficial digital flexor tendon, probably subcutaneous oedema. There is a subtle area of decreased echogenicity in the centre of the superficial digital flexor tendon. (b) There is a suspicion of damage of the superficial digital flexor tendon. The horse should be restricted to box rest for 10–14 days and re-evaluated. There seems to be variability between horses as to when a lesion is best identified ultrasonographically relative to the onset of clinical signs and caution must always be exercised when examining a horse in the most acute phase.

The horse was treated as advised and the heat and pain disappeared, but a follow-up ultrasonographic examination revealed a much more obvious area of reduced echogenicity within the superficial digital flexor tendon (*Figure 300*). It should also be noted in the follow-up ultrasonogram that although the gain settings are similar to those of the previous scan (the deep digital flexor tendon is of similar echogenicity in each), the palmar aspect of the superficial digital flexor tendon is diffusely hypoechoic.

241 Although haematology and blood biochemistry may be helpful in the assessment of neonatal septicaemia, results can be equivocal. However, measurement of serum IgG to evaluate the adequacy of passive transfer of immunity would be essential in a case like this. Serum or plasma IgG can be measured in several different ways. These may include measurement of total protein, the zinc sulphate turbidity test, coated latex bead agglutination, enzyme-linked immunosorbent assay (ELISA) and radial immunodiffusion. All of these methods have inherent problems and there are differences of opinion as to the level of IgG that represents failure of passive transfer. Some reports have suggested that < 400 mg/dl of IgG at 24 h post partum may be inadequate and others prefer to see levels of > 800 mg/dl. Such debate may not be appropriate when the clinician is presented with a foal that is weak and cold that is the produce of a dam that has 'run-milk' prior to foaling or is producing little if any milk at all. Plasma transfusion would be necessary if failure or passive transfer has occurred, and under these circumstances it is reasonable to try to attain an IgG level of at least > 400 mg/dl by the administration of at least 1 l of plasma by slow intravenous transfusion.

Blood culture may also be helpful in these circumstances, so that bacterial sensitivity can be established. It is preferable to obtain blood cultures after thorough preparation of the collection site by sterile needle venepuncture, rather than through a catheter. At least 10 ml of blood should be withdrawn from the vein and the collection needle should be discarded and replaced with a further sterile needle before placing the sample in the blood culture bottle(s).

242 (a) Cystic calculus.
(b) Calcium carbonate (calcium oxalate, magnesium, ammonium, phosphate).
(c)
• Cystotomy via a ventral paramedian incision.

- Pararectal cystotomy.
- Ischial urethrostomy ± crushing with a lithotrite or electrohydraulic lithotripsy.
(d)
- Cystotomy – peritonitis, bladder leakage, incisional infection, wound dehiscence.
- Ischial urethrostomy – urethral trauma, urethral stricture, urethral fistula, increased incidence of recurrence.

243 (a) Lethal white foal (resulting from the breeding of two overo paints) is the most likely diagnosis. The primary lesion is ileocolonic aganglionosis, with or without intestinal stenosis or agenesis. Retained meconium should be considered.
(b) A conclusive ante-mortem diagnosis is difficult to achieve. The signals (white colour, breeding and clinical course) are strongly suggestive. A simple meconium impaction should be ruled out. Abdominal radiographs may be supportive of the diagnosis. A positive contrast study may be helpful.
(c) There is no treatment.

244 (a) Diabetes insipidus. This condition arises due to failure of antidiuretic hormone (ADH) to affect the collecting ducts of the kidney. Diabetes insipidus may be classified as either central, due to insufficient output of ADH from the pituitary gland, or nephrogenic, due to failure of the collecting ducts to respond to ADH. Animals with either form of diabetes insipidus cannot concentrate urine following a water-deprivation test.
(b) Yes. A water-deprivation test is contraindicated in an azotaemic animal because renal failure could be exacerbated by dehydration. This pony had normal plasma creatinine and urea concentrations, although these do not entirely exclude renal disease since they are relatively insensitive indicators of glomerular infiltration rate. However, in this case the duration of clinical signs was chronic such that if the excessive thirst had been a result of primary renal disease there would be changes in plasma creatinine or urea.
(c) ADH response test. The suggested test protocol is three injections of 60 iu ADH/450 kg at intervals of 6 h. Following these injections a case of central diabetes insipidus will be able to concentrate urine, whereas one of renal origin still produces dilute urine.

245 In the non-pregnant mare, fluid in the uterus should be viewed with suspicion. In early oestrus the presence of some clear black fluid is probably normal (see *Figure 298P*), but its accumulation may reflect an impaired ability of the uterus to drain fluid efficiently. After ovulation and in dioestrus, especially in mares which have been covered, fluid in the uterus usually indicates an exudate resulting from a bacterial endometritis (*Figure 301A* – note that the fluid is not completely clear). In mid or prolonged dioestrus, uterine fluid (exudate) may become very echodense (concentrated) and difficult to differentiate from uterine tissue (*Figure 301B*). *Figure 301C* shows a normal dioestrus uterus (above the arrows) on top of the bladder; the latter contains echodense urine with some clearer (black) pockets.

246
- The repair must be performed under general anaesthetic.
- Prepare routinely the area for aseptic surgery.
- Elevate the mucosa from the skin gum margin and from the free lower lip.
- Place both resectioned areas together to ensure all areas of future contact have

subcutaneous contact.
- Suture the inside mucous membrane of the gum and lip with single interrupted sutures using a non-absorbable material, e.g. polypropylene.
- Then suture the outside skin and subcutaneous tissue with single interrupted sutures.
- Support the weight of the lower lip by large horizontal mattress sutures across the commissure.
- Restrict lip movement by support with elastoplast around the nose and lower lip.
- Tube feed with gruel for 2 weeks to allow healing.

247 (a) Autonomic ganglia – cranial cervical, stellate, ganglia of the sympathetic trunk or coeliacomesenteric ganglia.
(b) This section of stellate ganglion shows loss of basophilic Nissl substance; pyknosis, margination and loss of nuclei; multiple, small vacuoles in the cytoplasm.
(c) These findings are typical of acute and subacute grass sickness.

248 (a) The blood picture suggests a protein-losing gastroenteropathy. The rectal biopsy indicates colitis, but the poor glucose tolerance test points to quite severe intestinal disease. Although the nodules palpated per rectum could be lymph nodes, they could also be neoplastic, and one could reasonably surmise that this is a possible lymphosarcoma case. This was confirmed at post-mortem (*Figure 302A* and *B*).
(b) Chronic weight loss with or without diarrhoea demands a systematic and thorough work-up. The owner should be warned of the expense and the possibility of failure to diagnose or successfully treat the condition.
  (i) History: check worming programme, dental care, quality of feed and conditions of feeding (e.g. competition for food), pasture management, work programme and housing.
 (ii) Physical examination should be as exhaustive as possible. Bear in mind that weight loss can be caused by tooth problems, parasites, disease of the alimentary tract, the respiratory tract, the liver, the urinary tract, the cardiovascular system and the reproductive tract; chronic pain or chronic infection. More than one system may be involved.
(iii) Laboratory tests. In this case your physical examination suggests gastrointestinal disease, but this can always be accompanied by liver disease. Do a basic screening first:
- Full haematology. Anaemia common. WBC often normal.
- Proteins, including electrophoresis for globulin fractions; may distinguish liver disease, parasite damage and bacterial infections.
- Enzymes AST, SDH, GGT, bilirubin, IAP.
- Faeces. Parasitology and bacteriology. Should repeat several times.
- Peritoneal fluid. Usually negative in lymphosarcoma and chronic bowel wall disease.
Evaluate these then proceed to:
- Glucose tolerance test.
- Rectal biopsy.
Further possibilities:
- Ultrasonography.
- Laparoscopy.
- Laparotomy.

249 (a) A triangular opacity superimposed on the soft tissues plantar to the hock.
(b) The opacity was further investigated ultrasonographically. There was a triangular hyperechoic structure within a fluid-filled cavity in the soft tissues on the plantar aspect of the hock.
(c) Surgical exploration and removal of the foreign body. In this case it was a triangular piece of glass located in a small cavity filled with serous fluid on the edge of the plantar ligament.

250 (a) Rupture of the chordae tendineae of the right commissural cusp of the mitral valve.
(b) These cases often have a sudden onset of respiratory distress due to the development of pulmonary oedema. Auscultation in all cases would reveal a cardiac murmur of severe mitral regurgitation. The murmur would be pansystolic with the point of maximum intensity over the left hemithorax at the level of the mitral valve. The murmur would tend to radiate over a large area primarily dorsally and caudally. A precordial thrill would be palpable over the mitral area. A pansystolic murmur is often heard over the right hemithorax due to the referral of sound from the mitral regurgitation or due to the development of tricuspid regurgitation secondary to pulmonary hypertension and right ventricular dilatation. The third heart sound may be pronounced due to the increased flow during rapid filling. The heart rate will vary depending on the ability of the heart to adapt to the abnormal flow. In some cases the heart rate may be irregular because atrial fibrillation is present.
(c) The prognosis is poor, and will depend on the severity of the mitral regurgitation and the ability of the heart to compensate for the abnormal flow. In most cases the regurgitation will be sufficiently severe to limit performance and most cases will develop congestive cardiac failure.

251 Although melanomas are common in the perineal region of the horse, the next most common general area for their occurrence is in the parotid region. The lesions at this site are secondary tumour deposits within lymphoid tissue. The most likely site for primary melanoma formation is in the submucosa of the auditory tube diverticulum (ATD) (guttural pouch). Ectopic melanosis can be found in the ATDs in 60% of grey horses, and the usual location is in the lateral compartment adjacent to the internal maxillary vessels. A primary melanoma can always be found at this site (*Figure 303*) in horses with external evidence of melanoma formation in the parotid glands.

252 (a) The clinical findings are highly suggestive of neoplasia. Abdominal masses in adult horses usually represent either tumours or abscesses. The absence of neutrophilia in either the blood or the peritoneal fluid suggests that the mass is not an abscess; malignant cells are only infrequently found in peritoneal fluid samples from cases of neoplasia. The history of recurrent bouts of choke suggests a partial obstruction of the oesophagus or cardia by tumour. The most common tumours to present in this form are lymphosarcoma and gastric squamous cell carcinoma.
(b) The precise diagnosis can only be made by histological examination of biopsy material obtained by exploratory laparotomy or possibly by percutaneous, ultrasound-guided biopsy. Gastric lavage may sometimes yield exfoliated malignant cells in cases of gastric squamous cell carcinoma; gastroscopy may also enable direct visualisation and biopsy of tumour masses in the stomach. Radiography of the thorax might reveal evidence of neoplasia in the chest.

253 (a) The rounded fragment present in the distal tarsocrural (tibiotarsal) joint indicates that the hock problem is chronic in nature. Therefore, it is not related to the mandibular fracture.
(b) Osteochondrosis dissecans of the distal aspect of the lateral trochlear ridge of the talus (tibial tarsal) bone.
(c) The tarsocrural effusion usually responds well to surgical treatment of the osteochondrosis lesion, by curettage of the abnormal part of the parent bone and removal of separate fragments.

254 (a) Microsporosis (spread by biting fly, *Stomoxys*).
(b) Rubbing, contact with infected gear, horse transporters, soil, or infection from biting arthropods, such as mosquitoes or *Stomoxys calcitrans*.
(c) *Microsporum gypseum* can live as a soil saprophyte, on contaminated brushes and walls of stables, and in horse transporters.

255 (a) An apparently icteric sclera is present. The sign may have marked or no clinical significance!
(b) The presence of this sign alone may be due to the ingestion of a diet with a high carotene content (such as green grass) or may arise from a period of inappetence. Possible causes of inappetence should be identified. Icterus associated with pyrexia and/or anaemia is very significant and conditions such as equine infectious anaemia, babesiosis, leptospirosis and other haemolytic disorders should be considered. Significant icterus may arise from biliary obstruction or from hepatic disease (such as plant poisonings, etc.).

256 No, this is certainly not the typical appearance of mycosis in the auditory tube diverticulum. The view shows the roof of the right medial compartment with the tympanic bulla centrally, the head of the styloid process of the hyoid to the left and the internal carotid artery to the right of the photograph. More rostrally there appear to be areas of submucosal haemorrhage but no mycotic plaque is visible. An oral inspection shows multiple submucosal haemorrhages (*Figure 304*). This is a case of immune-mediated thrombocytopenia (IMTP).
It is likely that the IMTP in the case described was drug induced and related to the antimicrobial therapy employed to treat the sinusitis. The mare was not anaemic and therefore whole blood transfusions were not required but these may be needed if severe anaemia is present. In any event the haematocrit should be monitored during the recovery period. The antibiotic treatment should be withdrawn or at least changed to a chemically dissimilar agent. Most horses with IMTP respond well to corticosteroid therapy.

257 (a) Squamous cell carcinoma.
(b) Histopathological examination.
(c) Excision of the nictitating membrane, followed by careful examination of the rest of the conjunctiva for evidence of spread. If necessary, β-irradiation.

258 (a) At least within the first 12 h post partum, preferably within the first 6 h.
(b) The consistency is sticky, and the colour varies. The best way to assess quality is with a colostrometer that measures specific gravity.
(c) For good passive transfer of antibodies, at least 1 l of colostrum with specific gravity > 1.060 is suggested.

(d) Most normal Thoroughbred foals consume 125–150 kcal/kg/day. For this size foal, this caloric intake can be provided by approximately 12 l of goat's milk, at about 500 ml/kg/h. Minimum requirements to maintain adequate hydration are estimated at 80–100 ml/kg/day.
(e) This varies with geographical location and the circumstances at the farm. Nurse mares are probably the best choice. A variety of commercially available milk replacers are now available.
(f) Weight gain (normal Thoroughbred foals gain 1–2 kg/day); urine specific gravity (usually < 1.010 in healthy, normally nursing foals); add up total intake over a 24-h period.
(g) Treat with tetanus antitoxin, dip umbilicus with antiseptic, and quantitate IgG level at 18 h of age; possibly use an enema. Perhaps measure complete blood count and fibrinogen.

259 Mares which are barren at the end of the breeding season should be examined for persistent endometritis and treated as necessary. They (and if possible maiden mares) should then be turned out to rough off in the early winter, during which they may lose weight; they should be inspected occasionally to ensure that they do not start aspirating air into the vagina.

The mares should then be housed from early December and given hard feed. From mid-December at the latest they should be subjected to at least 16 h good light a day. The quality of light is important and it should illuminate the whole of the stable to such an extent that it is possible to read a newspaper, even in the corners and outside the door, if the mare is able to put her head out.

By mid-February some mares will be losing their winter coats and will be cycling. Those which have follicular activity that is judged insufficient to lead to imminent ovulation may be treated with a progestogen to try to stimulate an early luteal phase. Allyltrenbolone is usually administered in the food for 10–14 days, although an intravaginal progesterone-releasing device (marketed for use in cattle) has also been used. These drugs suppress the release of luteinising hormone (LH) from the pituitary gland, thus encouraging an accumulation of the hormone for subsequent release. Follicle-stimulating hormone (FSH), however, continues to be released and causes continued growth of follicles to + 2 cm diameter; larger follicles are occasionally seen at this time. FSH is normally responsible for the follicular growth that occurs during the luteal phase of the cycle. LH causes both maturation of follicles during the long oestrus of the mare and subsequent ovulation. In many cases, withdrawal of the progesterone is therefore followed by an ovulatory oestrus.

Gonadotrophin-releasing hormone (GnRH) has also been used to induce ovulation early in the year. Experimentally, subcutaneous devices which are capable of releasing this hormone in small doses over prolonged periods have been used successfully; they are not available commercially. Twice daily administration of GnRH to mares which have some initial follicular development may stimulate an ovulation. However, should the mare fail to conceive it is likely that she will return to anoestrus.

The use of eCG in this situation is completely ineffectual because the blood concentrations which occur during normal pregnancy cannot be achieved using the products available.

Note: Anticipation of an ovulatory oestrus early in the year, using thorough examination with either palpation or ultrasonography, is one of the most difficult clinical judgements that has to be made with broodmares. It is often necessary to examine the mare frequently during the transition from anoestrus to ovulation, a dilemma not usually appreciated by the mare's owner.

260 (a) Chronic renal failure (CRF). The diagnosis is made on the basis of laboratory evidence of azotaemia, hypercalcaemia, hypophosphataemia, hyponatraemia and hypochloraemia together with anaemia.

The finding of hypercalcaemia and hyperphosphataemia in advanced renal failure in the horse is a species peculiarity for which the reason is unknown.

Other blood biochemical abnormalities detected in some case of equine CRF include hypoproteinaemia, hyperkalaemia and hyperlipidaemia.

Polydipsia and polyuria are not consistently present in CRF in the horse. Additional clinical signs which may develop in some cases are peripheral oedema and oral ulceration.

(b) Equine CRF usually arises due to chronic interstitial nephritis, which may be a sequel to a variety of renal conditions, most commonly acute renal failure due to either shock (e.g. hypovolaemia, endotoxaemia) or following toxicities (e.g. aminoglycoside antibiotics, non-steroidal anti-inflammatory drugs, myoglobin pigment).

Renal or ureteral calculi may result in equine CRF directly by obstructing urinary flow (leading to hydronephrosis) or indirectly, by causing chronic interstitial nephritis. Conversely, nephroliths may arise as a consequence of mineralising interstitial fibrosis and/or the abnormal urinary excretion of minerals in equine CRF.

The coexistence of pyelonephritis and renal calculi in the horse is not uncommon. Pyelonephritis *per se* may give rise to interstitial fibrosis.

Glomerulonephritis can commonly be identified in the horse at post-mortem examination but this condition is not commonly associated with clinical renal disease.

Renal neoplasia occurs uncommonly in the horse and affected animals generally do not have either clinical or laboratory findings of renal failure although they will develop signs of progressive weight loss ± anorexia ± abdominal pain ± haematuria.

261 (a) There is facial swelling with palpebral oedema and filling of the supraorbital fossae. The oral mucous membranes are congested and the tongue shows petechial haemorrhages.

(b) African horse sickness is the most likely diagnosis. It occurs in areas of Africa, the Middle East and Southern Europe.

(c) The disease is transmitted by biting insects (particularly *Culicoides*) and has a marked seasonality associated with the presence of the vector. Dogs, wild equids and possibly other animals may act as reservoirs of infection. Vaccinated or previously challenged animals may be immune or may be affected by a mild infection in which a short-lived fever and slight respiratory tract signs may be present. Totally susceptible horses may die within 12–48 h. Control by vaccination is widely practised. Control of the vector is probably impossible and it is impractical to protect the horses from vector challenge.

262 (a)
• A previous subsolar abscess which has discharged at the coronary band.
• Sole bruising. The wet ground may cause the sole to soften, predisposing to bruising.
• Stake wound. This is less likely, as the discharge is below the coronary band.
• Coronitis. This is unlikely since there is not sufficient true skin involvement.
(b)
• If the lameness is only due to bruising, the horse may respond if confined to a dry

stable for a few days.
- If there is no improvement, or if there is subsolar abscess, cut out the affected sole, flush out the sinus with hydrogen peroxide and/or metronidazole many of the infecting organisms are anaerobes). If a large area of sole is removed it may be helpful to apply a shoe with a screw-on boiler plate, which can be removed to facilitate subsequent treatment, but provides protection to exposed sensitive tissues.

263 (a) An incomplete condylar fracture of the left third metacarpal bone spiralling proximally from the fetlock joint. The nature of the fracture would suggest that this is a medial condylar fracture, as was the case, although this is not obvious from the radiograph.
(b) The classic condylar fracture of the third metacarpal bone is the lateral condylar fracture in the racehorse, which tends to course proximolaterally and may become complete on the lateral aspect of the bone. It does not normally spiral, as is the case with medial condylar fractures. It is very important to examine radiographically the entire length of the bone.
(c) Either casting or lag screw fixation following the spiral of the fracture so that at each level the screws are at 90° to the fracture plane. In contrast to the lateral condylar fracture, it may be necessary to insert screws along the whole length of the metacarpus.

264 (a) *Figure 203A* is a lateromedial view. There is a relatively lucent area in the distal dorsal aspect of the distal phalanx. The lucent zone is sharply delineated and appears to penetrate the dorsal cortex of the bone. There is slight separation in the dorsal wall up to the level of the lesion in the distal phalanx. There is a radiopaque arrow on the solar surface of the foot.
Figure 203B is a dorsoproximal–plantarodistal oblique view. There is an extremely well-circumscribed, approximately circular lucent zone in the distal aspect of the distal phalanx. The surrounding bone appears to be normal.
(b) Keratoma, other non-neoplastic mass, osseous cyst-like lesion, other tumour, result of previous infection.
(c) Surgical exploration: a dorsal approach is recommended in this case.
A partial dorsal hoof wall resection was performed and an extremely well-circumscribed spherical soft-tissue mass was removed. Histological examination revealed a non-neoplastic epidermal inclusion cyst.
(d) If a keratoma or non-neoplastic mass, good.

265 (a) 4–5 l, based on a dehydration estimate of 8–10% of body weight.
(b) 80–100 ml/kg body weight, or 4–5 l/24-h period.
(c) Intravenous replacement solution, such as Plasmalyte or lactated Ringers, with potassium supplemented (because of hypokalaemia, acidosis, and continuing losses of K^+). Depending on the foal's blood glucose, and whether the foal begins to suckle, a continuous glucose infusion may also be indicated. Oral glucose–electrolyte solutions may be provided.
(d) Part of a generalized infection; enteropathogenic *E. coli*, *Salmonella*, *Actinobacillus*, Rotavirus-induced diarrhoea.
(e) Broad-spectrum antibiotics, bismuth subsalicylate, nutritional support, possibly plasma (if low IgG concentration), possibly anti-ulcer medication.

266 (a) Fractured sacrum and polyneuritis equi are the two diseases most likely to cause such a profound example of the cauda equina syndrome.

(b) Rectal examination and cranial nerve examination. Quite frequently a rectal examination allows palpation of a fracture site or a fracture callus on the floor of the sacrum, usually at the region of S2. With polyneuritis equi there is very frequently involvement of cranial nerves, particularly V, VII and VIII, and evidence for this must be searched for.

267 (a) The absorptive phase of the response is affected by the rate of gastric emptying, mucosal cell function, intestinal transit time and previous dietary history.
(b) The absorption response in this animal shows a delayed peak at 180 min rather than 120 min. This suggests either a reduced rate of gastric emptying or a reduced intestinal transit time. The history of recurrent bouts of abdominal pain associated with feeding suggests the presence of a gastric or partial small intestinal obstruction (e.g. tumour).

268 (a) The horse has pale mucous membranes, suggestive of anaemia. Equine infectious anaemia (EIA) (swamp fever) and lymphosarcoma are commonly associated with an intermittent fever over the time course (3 months) indicated. Anaemia is invariably present with EIA and may be seen in association with lymphosarcoma either due to anaemia of chronic disease or associated with red blood cell haemolysis.
(b) As lymphosarcoma is unlikely to affect more than one horse, EIA should be considered.
(c) Coggin's test (agar gel immunodiffusion) is routinely used to detect carriers and recovered horses. There is a very high incidence of carrier animals and the disease is probably transmitted by biting insects, but iatrogenic transmission is relatively easy. Coggin's test is, however, extremely effective and has been responsible for accurate detection of infected and recovered animals. Control of vectors or the isolation of horses from the vectors are probably impractical measures under most circumstances.

269 There are two abnormalities which should be noted:
- Asymmetry of the rima glottidis due to left recurrent laryngeal neuropathy (RLN). The left arytenoid cartilage (right in *Figure 207*) is hanging towards the midline.
- The horse has been subjected to previous surgery which has consisted of ventriculocordectomy on the left side. Note loss of the sharp edge of the vocal cord and the white scar tissue in the normal purple recess of the ventricle. There has possibly been ventriculectomy on the right. The latter is not clear from *Figure 207*.

Was the purchaser aware that the horse had been subjected to previous surgery? If not, there would probably be grounds in civil law for the sale to be revoked and/or for the purchaser successfully to claim for any loss sustained in transportation costs, etc. Horses sold at auction with evidence of RLN, particularly when previous surgery has not been declared, are usually returnable to the vendor under the Conditions of Sale. When there is the slightest possibility of a dispute, it is imperative that the veterinary surgeon makes full notes, which, in this case, should include:
- Date, time and venue of examination.
- Formal identification of horse.
- External evidence of RLN:
  – palpable evidence of laryngeal muscle atrophy;
  – response to slap test.
- Evidence of previous surgery, i.e. palpable laryngotomy cicatrix.
- Details of endoscopic findings.
- Result of exercise test – what adventitious respiratory sounds could be heard?

Alternatively, if the horse was acquired by a purchaser who was aware of the history of laryngeal disease, advice may be sought on possible treatment, depending on the athletic expectations of the animal. Although it is recognised that prosthetic laryngoplasty ('tie-back') surgery can produce occasional complications in the forms of coughing or nasal reflux of ingesta, the risks are justifiable in a horse which is otherwise an ineffective athlete.

270 (a)
- Preservation of blood supply to the avulsed skin flap.
- Using a sterile gloved hand, determination of the extent of the wound and possible injury to the associated bones, joints, tendons and tendon sheaths. A radiographic examination would also be applicable.
- Initial irrigation/lavage of the wound to reduce contamination.
- Immobilisation and support of the limb using splints, and a Robert–Jones bandage.
- This animal has sustained a considerable injury to the left forelimb. Are there any systemic signs that predisposed to this traumatic incident, e.g. evidence of abdominal colic or neurological disease? What other injuries have been sustained, e.g. abdominal wall/diaphragmatic/bladder rupture, other limb or head and neck injuries?
- Has there been a significant blood loss? – evidenced by pale mucous membranes, low PCV or tachycardia.

(b)
- Blood supply to the skin flap.
- Presence of devitalised tissue.
- Wound contamination – less than 10^6 organisms/g of tissue is compatible with healing but is dependent on the tissue damage and type of bacterial inoculum.
- Seroma/haematoma formation beneath the skin flap resulting in separation of the tissue surfaces. (Formation of dead space.)
- Presence of sequestra or foreign bodies.
- Movement of tissue surfaces over the carpus.
- Correct choice and use of suture material.
- Nutritional status of the animal, total plasma proteins greater than 6 g/dl.
- Soft tissue/bony damage distal to this wound.

(c)
- Debridement – surgically and by wound lavage using antiseptic solutions.
- Mesh expansion.
- Use of passive or active (suction) drains to reduce dead space.
- Correctly applied bandage or cast to reduce oedema, haematoma formation, protection against further damage or contamination. Immobilisation of the limb and absorption of exudate from the wound surface.
- Antibiosis and analgesia.

271 (a) Chronic laminitis.
(b) Chronic laminitis may be a sequel to acute laminitis due to grain overload, excessive consumption of rich grass, etc. It may also be the result of poor foot care; originally, proper trimming would have prevented this condition from deterioration.
(c) The feet should be radiographed (lateromedial views) in order to establish the degree of rotation of the distal phalanges, and any secondary changes which may have developed which may influence the long-term prognosis for return to full athletic function. Careful corrective trimming and shoeing should result in dramatic

improvement within 3–6 months. In selected cases the use of a heart bar shoe may improve the comfort of the patient.

272 (a) The horse is suffering from idiopathic postoperative paralytic ileus (absence of coordinated gastrointestinal activity). Ileus can also be secondary to localised peritonitis, adhesions, mechanical obstruction or gut infarction. However, in these cases gut sounds tend to persist longer, the rise in PCV is slower and delayed in onset and signs of abdominal discomfort are usually more pronounced. Postoperative paralytic ileus is a major case of death following abdominal surgery.
(b) Factors predisposing to postoperative paralytic ileus appear to be:
- Gut ischaemia.
- Bowel distension.
- Surgical handling.
- Endotoxaemia.

However, it does not seem possible to predict individual susceptibility to ileus based on these criteria.
(c) An attempt to treat postoperative paralytic ileus should include:

- The administration of non-steroidal anti-inflammatory drugs (NSAIDs) to protect the bowel wall against the endotoxins that induce ileus.
- Intravenous fluid administration to correct fluid loss and electrolyte imbalances and improve the microcirculation at the level of the bowel wall.
- Regular nasogastric intubation to achieve decompression of the stomach, relieve discomfort and avoid gastric rupture.
- Until recently no accepted pharmacological treatment existed for postoperative ileus. However, the use of the new prokinetic agent cisapride, administered at 8-hourly intervals following surgery, has been highly effective in reducing the incidence of idiopathic postoperative paralytic ileus.

(d) If the paralytic ileus proves refractory to medical therapy, repeated laparotomy and decompression of the small bowel by milking its contents into the caecum should be considered.
    Criteria for surgical intervention are:
- Increasing heart rate over 60–80 beats/min.
- Absence of peristaltic sounds.
- PCV over 50% despite fluid therapy.
- Continuous gastric reflux.
- Rectal evidence of significant small intestinal distension.

273 (a) Degenerative joint disease of the right coxofemoral joint, with marked modelling of the acetabulum.
(b) No treatment is possible so, unless the owner wants to retain the animal as a pet, euthanasia is indicated.

274 A Bromsulphlein (BSP) retention test and a liver biopsy may be helpful. BSP is a dye that is excreted by the liver. The test is based on the assessment of the amount of the dye that is excreted over a given time period. The 'half-life' is then calculated. Extended 'half-life' clearances are seen in the presence of gross hepatic malfunction.
    The jugular veins are prepared as for surgery. An initial (time 0) jugular venous serum sample (red-stoppered vacuum container) is collected. One gram of BSP is sufficient for a normal adult horse. This can usually be administered from two vials of the

commercially prepared reagent. This reagent must be prewarmed to body temperature before use, and then injected intravenously into the right jugular vein. Serum samples should then be collected (red-stoppered vacuum containers) from the opposite (left) jugular vein at 2, 4, 8 and 16 min after administration.

Liver biopsy is of value when serum biochemistry results indicate the presence of hepatic pathology. An imaginary straight line should be drawn, on the right side of the horse, from the shoulder joint to the point of the hip. The site for biopsy is in the space between the fourteenth and fifteenth ribs that is transected by the above line. This site is prepared as for surgery, with local anaesthesia of the skin and intercostal muscles. A stab incision is made in the skin with a sterile scalpel blade. A sterile 'Tru-cut' 6 in (12 cm) long biopsy needle is introduced at a 90° angle through the incision. The biopsy sample is then withdrawn, carefully removed from the needle to avoid artefacts, and placed in 10% formol saline.

Centrilobular damage to hepatocytes can occur (rarely) in horses that have had problems related to halothane anaesthesia.

275 (a) It is most likely that the lesions appeared at the time of the eruption of the permanent cheek teeth. They may be very unsightly but are rarely of clinical significance.
(b) The owner should be assured that they are of little importance unless associated with heat and pain. Lesions which are present in older horses will be even less likely to be of any importance and no treatment is either available or justified.
(c) The presence of a discharging sinus, heat, pain and swelling with local oedema indicate that the lesion is of possible significance, but in the absence of these symptoms another cause for the dysphagia should be sought.

276 (a) In most cases pregnancy can be diagnosed accurately at this time. The conceptus (vesicle) is black (fluid filled) and spherical, or may be slightly flattened dorsoventrally. There are white spots or lines on the dorsal and ventral surfaces of the conceptus, caused by intense echoes at the tissue/fluid boundaries. Often it is the presence of these lines that first indicate that the mare is pregnant. The conceptus can be anywhere in the uterus, so that a thorough search must be made; pregnancies at the tips of uterine horns can be missed, as can those at the base of the horns in an old mare with a pendulous uterus. Sequential scanning will reveal that up to the sixteenth day the conceptus is mobile in the uterus. *Figure 305A* shows a round 14-day conceptus in a uterine horn.
(b) From the sixteenth day the conceptus becomes 'fixed' at the base of one of the uterine horns; there is no relationship between the location of the conceptus and the side of ovulation. It is now 1.8–2.2 cm in diameter and still roughly spherical. Thereafter the conceptus continues to grow in this position. By the eighteenth day it is 2–3 cm in diameter and may be irregular in outline; 'corrugations' may occur on the dorsal surface and the conceptus may become markedly compressed dorsoventrally (*Figure 305B*).
(c) By 21 days the conceptus has grown little since 18 days; may still be irregular in outline and is often almost triangular in shape. By this time there is usually a small (1.5–2.0 mm) white dot on the periphery of the growing conceptus; this appears in the 4–8 o'clock position if the conceptus is viewed as a clock face. It is the embryo which is being lifted from the wall of the conceptus by the allantois developing beneath it. A feature of the uterus at this time is the thick and irregular dorsal wall compared with the thin ventral wall. This disparity in thickness may be responsible for the non-spherical shape of the conceptus at this time and could be the reason why the conceptus is

269

invariably aligned so that the embryo develops from the ventral surface. Embryos which develop on the dorsal surface have been known to result in viable foals. The 21-day pregnancy shown in *Figure 305C* appears smaller than at 18 days; this is because the embryo could not be imaged on the widest diameter of the conceptus.

(d) By 26 days the conceptus has increased slightly in size and the embryo is clearly separated from the ventral border of the conceptus by the allantois (*Figure 305D*). A white line to either side of the embryo is seen; this is the wall between dorsal yolk sac and ventral allantois. The embryonic heart beat is seen as a small black dot which flicks in and out of focus in the embryo. With 7.5-MHz transducers it can be detected as early as 23 days.

(e) By 30 days (*Figure 305E*) the developing ventral allantois is roughly the same volume as the dorsal yolk sac, which is becoming slightly smaller. The embryo is a central white elliptical/spherical structure, although its position can vary considerably – the allantois/yolk sac border is evident on both sides of the embryo and a heart beat is clearly seen. Sometimes the scanning plane is such that the yolk sac/allantois border appears vertical, i.e. running dorsoventrally.

(f) By 37 days the allantoic cavity is the major fluid compartment of the conceptus and the fetus (as it is now called because organogenesis is complete) is near the dorsal surface of the conceptus (*Figure 305F*). With higher frequency scanners parts of the amnion, which surround the fetus, may be seen at this time.

(g) With the diminishing size of the yolk sac, the walls between it and the allantois come together dorsal to the fetus. These membranes contain the mesodermally derived blood vessels which will become the umbilical arteries and veins. By 42 days the fetus is suspended, usually near the centre of the allantoic cavity, by the dorsally attached umbilical cord; the latter may contain a black (fluid-filled) cavity – the remnant of the yolk-sac (*Figure 305G*).

(h) By 60 days the fetus is usually lying on the ventral surface of the allantoic cavity, because the umbilicus has increased in length. If the long axis of the fetus is parallel to the ultrasound plane, an image resembling a fetus can be obtained. Usually, however, the fetus is perpendicular or tangential to the ultrasound plane, so that cross or oblique sections are obtained that appear circular or oval. Movement of the transducer laterally will allow the thorax (heart) to be located to confirm that the fetus is viable. At this time the dorsal wall of the conceptus, which had hitherto been smooth, becomes 'corrugated' due to foldings in the placental (allantoic/ endometrial) attachment (*Figure 305H*).

(i) By 100 days the pregnancy, which now occupies both the uterine horns and the body, has become too large to allow complete visualisation using 5-MHz and 7.5-MHz transducers. The dorsal wall of the uterus is even more convoluted than previously. A dorsoventral septum, which is probably part of the division between the uterine body and horn, may be imaged – this can be confused with the umbilical cord. Even with high frequency transducers, however, it is often possible to trap the fetus in one of the horns, which can be gently compressed to allow features of its anatomy to be identified. In particular, the heart, stomach, spinal cord, eye orbits and ribs can usually be seen. *Figure 305I* shows the ribs and spinal cord.

277 (a) Affected animals may show other abnormalities of micturition such as increased frequency of urination and/or adoption of posture of urination for prolonged periods.

Additionally, some animals may have mild, recurrent colic and/or loss of body condition and/or hindlimb stiffness.

Although urinary incontinence is a feature of horses with sabulous urolithiasis (as a consequence of urinary retention and overflow in those with bladder paralysis), generally animals with discrete calculi remain continent, but they may intermittently dribble urine.

(b) Cases presented with these signs are frequently diagnosed as cystitis on the basis of urinalysis findings and the presence of red and white blood cells and also bacteria. However, cystitis is considered to be a secondary effect of physical abrasion of the bladder mucosa in these cases, rather than the primary event which leads to the formation of the calculus.

Examination of the bladder via the rectum is possible in even small ponies and the presence of a cystic calculus can be readily appreciated as a firm, ovoid mass, usually situated ventrally within the cranial portion of the pelvic cavity.

Ultrasonography can also be used to confirm the diagnosis.

(c) Surgical removal of bladder calculi is usually performed via laparotomy in male horses, although techniques of pararectal cystotomy have been described.

In mares, cystotomy is not necessary since even large calculi can be removed via the urethral orifice. In some cases urethral sphincterectomy and/or fragmentation of the calculus *in situ* may be necessary prior to removal.

Postoperative management should include antibiotics for about 1 week. Dosing with ammonium chloride, at a daily dose rate of 20 mg/kg, as a urinary acidifier may be considered but the low palatability of this compound precludes its long-term use.

The prognosis for cases with discrete cystic calculi, such as that illustrated in *Figure 212*, is excellent.

278 (a) BSP is taken up by the liver from the blood, conjugated to glutathione and excreted in the bile; it can therefore be used to assess the functional capacity of the liver.
(b) The result gives insufficent evidence of impaired hepatic function. A $t_{1/2}$ exceeding 4 min is suspicious; over 5 min usually indicates significant hepatic disease.
(c) Hyperbilirubinaemia, alterations in blood flow due to hypovolaemia or severe gastrointestinal tract disturbances and impaired blood flow in the vein used for BSP administration may interfere with the results.

279 (a) Clearly, a cleft palate would be the most likely cause of dysphagia in a 1-day-old foal. An oral examination to confirm this diagnosis may be inconclusive because most clefts involve the midline of the soft palate and are invisible per os in the conscious animal. Endoscopy per nasum is the preferred technique, provided that a narrow instrument is available. Palatal defects in foals carry a poor prognosis because surgical corrections are radical and rarely successful.

Figure 306A shows a discrete congenital cyst of the palate which was causing severe obstruction of the larynx in the fashion of a ball valve. It also caused dysphagia. A lateral radiograph (*Figure 306B*) confirms the extent and site of the lesion in the other plane. The cyst was removed by a laryngotomy approach and the foal recovered uneventfully.
(b) Other causes of dysphagia in a young foal include congenital functional failures of the pharynx and oesophagus, cricopharyngeal aplasia, oesophageal stricture and even megoesophagus.

280 (a) Dermatophyte infection.
(b) Freshly plucked hairs from the peripheral edge of a fresh lesion.
(c) Sabouraud's agar at 25°C for 7–14 days. A negative result cannot be declared until

after at least 14 days.
(d)
● Fumigate all gear with formaldehyde gas.
● Treat affected area daily with:
   2.5% lime sulphur, 10% povidone–iodine, 0.3% Halamid
   (N-sodium-N-chloro-p-toluene sulphonamide) (chloramine) Wellcome Ringworm
   Ointment.
● Administer griseofulvin orally (in feed).

281 (a) There is modelling of the apex of the patella and fragmentation. This may be the result of previous trauma, osteochondrosis or a sequel to medial patellar desmotomy.
(b) If the horse was lame, associated with pain referrable to the femoropatellar joint, the joint should be explored surgically. No gait abnormality was noted in this case.

282 (a) Acute salmonellosis causes a severe colitis, sometimes with septicaemia. Endotoxaemia is a major pathological complication of salmonella colitis, and this has several important consequences, including fever, haemodynamic effects, leucopenia and leucocytosis, thrombocytopenia, hepatic effects and coagulopathies. The intense secretory response of the bowel also results in profound dehydration.
(b) Repeated clinical evaluations are important in monitoring the course of the disease and its response to treatment. Particular attention should be paid to the hydration status (skin turgor, capillary refill time, etc.), cardiovascular system (heart rate, peripheral pulse, etc.) and feet (for evidence of laminitis). Laboratory investigations should include the assessment of hydration (packed cell volume, total plasma protein) and severity of sepsis (total white cell count and differential cell count, plasma fibrinogen). Leucopenia and neutropenia are frequently observed early in the course of the disease; they are a result of endotoxaemia and in response to inflammatory mediators. Toxic changes in the leucocytes (especially neutrophils) are also sometimes observed. Horses with acute diarrhoea are typically hyponatraemic, hypochloraemic and hypokalaemic, and these serum electrolytes should be monitored (preferably daily). Renal function should be assessed by monitoring blood urea and creatinine; these parameters are often elevated due to dehydration and reduced renal perfusion. Acid–base balance should also be assessed if facilities for their measurement are available.

283 (a) The trace in *Figure 215* shows premature ventricular systoles. The P–R interval preceding the premature ventricular systole is short, the ventricular systole being unrelated to the atrial contraction. Where the group of premature ventricular systoles occurs, the P–R interval progressively shortens until the P-wave is buried in the premature R-wave.
(b) The premature waveforms in this lead are not very different from normal ventricular waveforms. This suggests that they may be junctional in origin.
(c) The clinical significance of premature ventricular complexes is difficult to ascertain. They can occur during infection, electrolyte imbalance, hypoxia and anaesthesia, but can also be indicative of myocardial disease. They can also be produced or suppressed by autonomic stimulation. Occasional premature ventricular complexes with no underlying cardiac abnormality are probably of little significance; however, a thorough cardiac examination and an assessment of the animal's response to exercise must be made. If secondary causes of premature ventricular systoles are ruled out, the presence of myocardial disease should be suspected. Premature complexes can disappear with

time and rest and subsequent re-examination is advisable. Sustained ventricular arrhythmias can have serious haemodynamic consequences. Ventricular premature complexes must be considered abnormal.

284 This is a so-called 'atheroma' of the false nostril. The lesion is, in fact, a sebaceous cyst which has developed from the glands in the lining of the false nostril and contains a paste-like grey secretion. These cysts do not generally intrude into the nasal airways and are asymptomatic. If removal is required for cosmetic reasons it is simply a matter of careful dissection. However, on no account should the nostril margin be transected; nor should the incision be transverse, for fear of damage to the nasolabialis muscle.

285 (a) It is likely that the crack has penetrated the sensitive laminae, causing pain when movement occurs.
(b) In some cases treatment is successful by cutting out the affected area from the coronet to the sole, placing transverse wire sutures and filling the defect with hoof acrylic. This treatment does not always work.
(c) The treatment is only permanent if the tear in the laminae heals; if it does not, then the crack will return once pressure is reapplied during work.
(d)
● Complete wall strip from 5–10 mm dorsal to the crack and from the sole to the coronet; apply either a three-quarter bar shoe or a three-quarter heart bar shoe and rest the horse until the lameness resolves.
● If lameness persists, a unilateral palmar digital neurectomy may have to be considered.

286 (a) This animal has a slight bilateral foreleg lameness which responds to palmar digital nerve blocks on at least one foot. A diagnosis of bilateral palmar foot pain can be made on clinical grounds; it may be associated with navicular disease.
(b) There is an oval lucency superimposed on the body of the navicular bone, suggestive of classic navicular disease. However, since the foot was not packed a palmaroproximal–palmarodistal oblique view was obtained to confirm the location of this lucency. This confirmed the lucency as a cyst in the body of the navicular bone.
(c) Navicular disease.

287 (a) Anthelmintic resistance of cyathostomes is a possible important consequence of this worming programme. Although resistance to phenothiazine and piperazine has been reported, generally the problem has been associated with benzimidazole compounds and usually there is side resistance between individual drugs of this group. When drugs of high efficacy are given frequently to a group of animals there is a strong 'selection pressure' for the development of anthelmintic resistance.
   This programme will not control bots in the animals but these parasites have only minor pathogenic significance.
(b) Evidence of clinical disease related to parasites would indicate a lack of efficacy of the worming programme, but this is an unreliable guide to the occurrence of anthelmintic resistance.
   The aim of any control programme is to minimise contamination of pasture with parasitic larvae. Pasture larval counts performed at regular intervals (4–6 weekly) throughout the grazing season in management situations of permanent grazing are a good method of monitoring the efficacy of worming programmes. Monitoring the faecal worm egg count (FWEC) of the grazing animals, preferably about 10–14 days following

anthelmintic dosing, is a useful method of assessing the efficacy of a worming programme. Positive FWECs at this time would be suggestive of anthelmintic resistance which should be further investigated by performing specific faecal egg count reduction (FECR) tests by measuring pre- and post-treatment FWECs. Ideally the test would include groups of positive (other anthelmintic) and negative (no anthelmintic) control animals.

Various *in vitro* tests for anthelmintic resistance are used in experimental studies, but these methods are not widely available for use in the field.

288 Although ultrasound examination has been responsible for a significant reduction in the number of pregnancies that are lost due to abortion of twins, it is likely that a few 'scanned' mares will still have twin pregnancies undiagnosed because:
- Fertilisation of two ova can occur up to 4 days or more apart. A single examination before the sixteenth day may then fail to detect the younger twin because it is less than 5 mm in diameter.
- Failure to scan the whole uterus, especially before day 16, may result in a second pregnancy being overlooked.
- Any factors which diminish the efficiency with which the mare can be examined, e.g. poor restraint, too much light on the VDU, will affect the accuracy of diagnosis.
- Between 18 and 23 days, unilateral twins may be missed because the scanning plane does not highlight the interconceptual membranes. Particularly irregular shaped pregnancies at this stage should be scanned carefully from side to side to try to identify any indication of a twin pregnancy. In cases of doubt a re-scan should be arranged, although in many cases this is impractical or too expensive.
- Triplets may be confused with twins.

289 (a) Neoplasia or inflammation.
(b) The most likely diagnosis is a sarcoid, due to the lesion's clinical appearance – a hard, non-painful swelling, involving the skin and free and movable from underlying parts.
(c) Biopsy for histopathological examination.

290 (a) Thyroid neoplasia. Equine thyroid adenomas occur commonly: they can usually be identified as small (3–4 cm) diameter, paralaryngeal swellings and generally they are not associated with clinical disease.

C-cell (parafollicular cell tumours and carcinomas of the equine thyroid are infrequently diagnosed.
(b) Histopathological examination of either surgical or transcutaneous biopsy specimens from the thyroid mass. (The lesion illustrated was confirmed as thyroid adenoma.) Equine thyroid tumours are usually non-functional so that measurement of thyroid hormones in blood from affected animals would not be helpful in diagnosis.
(c) In this case the size of the mass is large enough to give discomfort to the animal, so surgical excision is indicated, subject to physical evidence of the absence of metastases and pathological confirmation that the lesion is benign.

291 (a) A chip fracture of the dorsodistal aspect of the radial carpal bone.
(b) Arthroscopic removal of the fragment is the appropriate treatment. A full series of carpal radiographs should be obtained to ensure that there are no other lesions.

292 (a)
- Nodular necrobiosis.
- Nodular collagenolytic granuloma.
- Acute collagen necrosis.
- Eosinophilic granuloma.

(b) Calcareous deposits have occurred.

(c)
- Sublesional injection of corticosteroid (beware the skin may become thinner).
- Many to most nodules regress over a long period of time.
- Calcified nodules may have to be surgically excised.
- Some horses show improvement after repeated treatment with ivermectin.

293 (a) Bilateral epistaxis and swelling/oedema of the muzzle.
(b) Snake bite envenomation, purpura haemorrhagica, haemorrhagic diatheses associated with hepatic failure, disseminated intravascular (consumptive) coagulopathy. The latter disorders are not associated specifically with skin puncture wounds.
(c) Snake envenomation is unlikely to result in death as most bites transfer an insufficient quantity of venom to kill a horse, although in some areas of the world extremely dangerous snakes do exist. High mortality may be associated with many of the conditions in which haemorrhage and oedema are present. Haemorrhagic diatheses associated with severe hepatic failure and consumptive coagulopathy would invariably show other important signs, but purpura haemorrhagica may be difficult to confirm.

294 (a) Ultrasonographic examination of the plantar metatarsal soft tissues. Radiographic examination of the proximal metatarsus.
(b) In both the left and right hindlimbs the margins of the suspensory ligament are poorly defined. The ligament is enlarged in the median plane and is diffusely hypoechoic. In the right hindlimb there are focal areas of hyperechogenicity within the suspensory ligament. These features are consistent with proximal suspensory desmitis with probable areas of focal mineralisation within the right suspensory ligament.
(c) *Figure 225C* is a dorsoplantar projection. There is an ill-defined patchy increase in opacity of the proximal aspect of the third metatarsal bone, resulting in poor definition between the proximal subchondral bone plate and the underlying trabecular bone, laterally.

Figure 225 D is a lateromedial view. There is a well-circumscribed area of increased opacity on the plantar proximal aspect of the third metatarsal bone (large arrow) (*Figure 307*). This is probably enthesophyte formation (new bone formation at the site of ligamentous or tendinous attachments). There is increased opacity in the plantar subchondral bone (small arrows).
(d) Diagnosis: proximal suspensory desmitis.
Prognosis: poor, in view of the severity of the ultrasonographic abnormalities, their probable chronicity (in view of the presence of mineralisation), the presence of associated radiographic abnormalities and the conformation of the horse (straight hocks).

295 (a) A well-demarcated semicircular area of bone loss is present on the solar margin of the distal phalanx.
(b) A keratoma or other space-occupying lesion is causing pressure-induced bone resorption of the distal phalanx.
(c) Keratomas are often associated with persistent foot infection and slight lameness.

If the owner considers treatment is justified in this aged hunter, surgical removal of the whole of the keratoma is indicated.

296 (a) The National Research Council in America produces every few years *The Nutrient Requirements of Horses* (*see* National Research Council 1989). This may be too detailed for many owners but is a useful practice reference book although it is geared to American feeds and feeding practices. It provides background information on many topics; there is a useful section for determining individual requirements and it is accompanied by an IBM-compatible disc. One of the more current books dealing with just equine nutrition is *Equine Nutrition and Feeding* (Frape, 1986). A more recent book is *Horse Feeding and Nutrition*, 2nd edn (Cunha, 1991).
(b) In the UK, ADAS will provide advice on pasture management (building design, environmental aspects, etc.) via their equine advisors (contactable through area offices of ADAS). A book entitled *Pasture Management for Horses and Ponies* by McCarthy (1987) is available. Equine nutritionists (see (c) below) may also provide practical information.
(c)
- Many feed companies employ either full-time or consultant nutritionalists. (Many of the consultants will work independently as freelance consultants.) These people often have a great deal of practical experience designing feeding regimens, etc., and can be contacted via the companies concerned. This can be very valuable if nutritional questions arise whilst animals are fed a particular make of feed.
- ADAS will also provide information on all aspects of equine nutrition.
- There are a number of nutritionalists working independently of feed companies. They often write/advertise in the various equine journals.

(d) Good scientifically based nutritional information on the horse is very limited. Extrapolations often have to be made from other species, from ponies to horses, or recommendations are based on small numbers of animals or existing feeding regimens. This means that the conclusions reached are not necessarily scientifically valid. Therefore informed advice, based on current scientific knowledge and practical experience, may be preferable.

297 The wear pattern of the central incisors arose by abrasion and is highly suggestive that the horse is a crib-biter and/or wind-sucker. Although the vendor is responsible for any declaration that the horse is free from stable vices, the examining veterinary surgeon should ask the vendor directly whether the horse is known to crib or wind-suck. Regardless of the answer, he should observe the resting horse very carefully for any tendency to display these vices, and the client should be advised of the possible significance of the dental findings.

298 (a) Posterior luxation of the lens.
(b) A full assessment of the visual capacity of this and the other eye should be carried out before any rider is allowed to ride the horse. In the event that the other eye is normal, the animal may be capable of relatively normal work.

299 Red blood cell transfusion can become essential in cases of neonatal isoerythrolysis. Although thoroughly washed red blood cells obtained from the dam are the preferred option, geldings that have not received a blood transfusion can also be used as donors in these circumstances. Red blood cells can be separated from the whole blood collected into sterile transfusion packs in appropriately equipped laboratories.

Red blood cells can be permitted to settle under gravity where this service is not available. In either event, the plasma should be decanted and the red blood cells should be washed three times in sterile saline prior to transfusion.

It is usual to resuspend the washed red blood cells in a volume of normal saline that is equivalent to a PCV value of 70%. The total volume of blood that is required can be calculated from the formula:

$$\frac{\text{Body weight (kg)} \times \text{blood volume (ml/kg)} \times (\text{PCV desired} - \text{PCV observed})}{\text{PCV of donor or packed cells}}$$

The blood volume of neonatal foals can be assumed to be 150 ml/kg.
The foal should be muzzled for at least 24 h and offered an alternative milk source.

300 (i) *Pinch graft* – small pinch grafts 2–3 mm diameter are harvested from a donor site on the same horse and inserted into stab incisions (pockets) in the recipient graft bed. They are set in rows and the area is dressed with antibiotics; a sterile non-adherent pad is applied, followed by a sterile combined dressing and bandage.
- Advantage – can be done without general anaesthetic; reasonably good 'take'; does not need expensive equipment.
- Disadvantage – hair grows at all angles, cobblestone effect; poor quality skin often cracks and bleeds with movement.

(ii) *Pinch graft* – use of 7-mm biopsy punch to harvest graft aseptically and implant into 5-mm graft site; set in rows, bandage as above and bandage is left in place for 5–15 days, depending on exudation.
- Advantage – same as pinch but there is a larger skin area in each graft; better cosmetic effect; higher survival rate.
- Disadvantage – need general anaesthetic; multidirectional hair growth; must have very good preparation of donor bed.

(iii) *Split-thickness mesh expansion graft* – use ventral abdominal skin, harvested with an electric dermatome; split by use of meshing instrument – first we have to align hair pattern with that of the leg, and, second, do *not* over expand the mesh; bandages may have to be changed more frequently.
- Advantage – flexible and can cover uneven areas; easy to apply; opening in graft allows escape of any discharges; can withstand some movement; small donor sites to cover larger wounds.
- Disadvantage – expensive equipment and general anaesthetic.

301 (a) To-and-fro (*Figure 230A*) and circle system (*Figure 230B*).
(b) *To-and-fro*
- Advantages:
  - Economy.
  - Carbon dioxide absorption.
  - Conservation of heat and water of respiration.
  - Facility to provide intermittent positive pressure ventilation.
- Disadvantages:
  - Cannot see if soda lime exhausted and so build up of CO_2.
  - Dead space increases with duration of anaesthesia as soda lime first exhausted from volume nearest animal.
- Risk of inhalation of dust from soda lime and resulting pneumonia.
- Bulk next to animal's head.

Circle system
- Advantages:
  - Advantages of to-and-fro.
  - Soda lime generally visible so colour changes can be easily appreciated.
  - Bulk of machine away from animal's head.
  - Soda lime not in close contact with the animal's respiratory tract.
- Disadvantages:
  - Expense.

302 This is a common reason to be asked to examine a mare; possible causes of non-oestrus detection are:
- Winter anoestrus; usually she will be in poor condition and still have a winter coat.
- The transition into the breeding season, which may in some mares last up to 2 or more months; physically, the mare is usually as for winter anoestrus above.
- Cyclic oestrus may have been missed because of poor teasing technique or because the mare failed to exhibit behavioural oestrus. The state of the tract will reflect the stage of the oestrous cycle.
- Prolonged dioestrus; a persistent corpus luteum is preventing a return to oestrus.
- Granulosa cell tumour.
- Turner's syndrome – chromosomal anomalies may result in the mare having non-functional ovaries of less than 0.5 cm diameter and a very hypoplastic tubular tract which is so thin walled that is difficult to palpate. This is obviously a condition of maiden mares and should be distinguished from the prepubertal condition which may still be seen in 2–4-year-old Thoroughbred fillies which have recently been in training.

303 (a) The radiograph appears to show a wing fracture of the distal phalanx, although a crimp mark partly overlying the heel of the shoe on this side of the film suggests that the wing fracture may be artefactual.
(b) A second view of the distal phalanx should be obtained, which in this case was normal. More importantly, radiographic investigation of the site of pain, the fetlock joint here, is indicated. This revealed an apical fracture of a sesamoid bone, indicating a severe injury to this joint in the past which was still causing the animal pain.

304 (a) Rectal examination should include a careful search for iliac thrombosis which is a possibility with this history, and for signs of bowel obstruction. Check for gastric reflux and if still in doubt about colic abdominal paracentesis may help. Examine the feet and digital pulses. Laminitis do not usually paw but acute traumatic laminitis is very painful and this should be considered. Pleurisy also causes colicky signs, so auscultation of the lungs should elucidate this. Palpate the back and hindlimb muscles. Take a blood sample for muscle enzymes as well as haematology. If the horse urinates and the urine is black, as it was with this horse, you are in luck! Even at this stage the CPK levels will be high and AST levels will rise over 24 h.
(b) This was a case of exertional rhabdomyolysis.
(c)
- Analgesia. Phenylbutazone intravenously is an effective treatment. Flunixin meglumine or butorphanol can also be used. Analgesia is vital since some severe cases become very distressed and this adversely affects their chance of recovery.
- Tranquillisers. Acetylpromazine is beneficial in improving peripheral blood flow but should not be used if there is any circulatory compromise. If necessary small doses of

xylazine or detomidine can be used.

- Corticosteroids improve tissue perfusion and stabilise cell membranes if administered in the first few hours.
- Fluid therapy is indicated in severe cases with myoglobinuria. Myoglobin is nephrotoxic and renal failure can be a fatal sequel in extreme cases. Give balanced electrolytes until the urine clears. These horses are usually alkalotic so do not give bicarbonate unless you have proved acidosis. Diuretics are contraindicated. Use the laboratory to assess progress and include blood urea nitrogen (BUN).
- Do not neglect good nursing. Examine the diet and electrolyte levels of recurrent cases.

305 (a) Several well-defined, encapsulated pulmonary abscesses with fluid lines can be seen.
(b) No!
(c) The most likely diagnosis is *Rhodococcus equi* abscessating bronchopneumonia. Culture of a tracheal aspirate is useful to confirm the infective organism. Other clinical signs may include a mild cough, tachypnoea, dyspnoea, poor growth and diarrhoea.
(d) A combination of erythromycin and rifampin.

306 (a) Head-pressing behaviour associated with hepatic encephalopathy.
(b) Two factors are thought to be involved – hyperammonaemia due to failure of the liver to convert ammonia to urea, and a decrease in the ratio of branched-chain to aromatic amino acids in the blood. The latter interferes with neurotransmitter activity in the CNS.
(c) Treatment involves oral administration of lactulose, which acidifies the colonic contents for conversion of ammonia to ammonium ions, which are not absorbed. Oral neomycin decreases ammonia production by intestinal bacteria but is of dubious value. Supplementation of the diet with branched-chain amino acids may be useful; sugar beet pulp is a good source.

307 (a) There is a diffuse increase in soft tissue opacity which has a nodular pattern.
(b) Examination of abdominal organs per rectum, abdominal ultrasonography, blood biochemistry/urinalysis, renal biopsy.
   The weight loss in this animal concurred with periodic haematuria, which, together with the radiological changes, were suggestive of a primary neoplasm of the urinary tract. Such tumours are uncommon with the exception of squamous cell carcinoma of the external genitalia. The diagnostic protocol in this case is directed towards the identification of a primary lesion by palpation and/or ultrasound imaging.
   The urinary bladder can be readily palpated per rectum, but only the caudal pole of the left kidney is palpable by this method such that it is not always possible to appreciate the presence of renal swelling or masses.
   The size, shape and internal structure of equine kidneys may be appreciated by ultrasonographic examination, and this method of investigation is of use in cases with suspected renal masses.
   In documented cases of renal neoplasia in the horse, the animals were often found to have normal values for blood biochemistry; non-specific haematological changes, e.g. neutrophilia, and analyses of urine simply confirmed haematuria, although in some cases neoplastic cells were evident on cytological examination of urinary sediment.
   Percutaneous renal biopsy may be undertaken in the horse but this procedure carries a high risk of haemorrhage such that it is inappropriate in most cases and is certainly

unnecessary in animals in which there is evidence of tumour metastasis.

At post-mortem examination of this case the radiological changes were found to represent pulmonary metastases of a renal adenocarcinoma.

308 (a)
- Allergy to feed, drugs, insects.
- Contact dermatitis.
- Purpura haemorrhagica.

(b)
- Antihistamines – tripelennamine 1 ml/40 kg.
- Corticosteroids – dexamethasone 3 mg/50 kg.
- Phenylbutazone – 1 g/200 kg daily.

(c)
- Would be unlikely if the exciting substance is not given again; i.e. penicillin or sulpha drugs.
- Feed-induced allergy does not appear to be easily reproduced.

309 (a) Carriers of *Salmonella* spp organisms are particularly liable to develop acute salmonellosis if they are subjected to significant stress (which may be relatively minor in extent). Any horse which subsequently develops an acute febrile diarrhoeic syndrome should be investigated carefully for the possibility of salmonellosis.
(b) Precautions should be taken immediately to protect people handling the animal or its contaminated bedding, etc. Isolation from other horses and the provision of foot baths and full hygiene controls should be instituted immediately. Rectal swabs should be taken on five or more consecutive days (and possibly a rectal biopsy) and cultured for *Salmonella* organisms. Although the animal may be acutely affected the organisms may be extremely difficult to isolate.
(c) Acute infections may result in a rapid death; pyrexia is suggestive of concurrent septicaemia. In the absence of septicaemia supportive fluid therapy may allow recovery of the horse. The prognosis should remain guarded. Recovered animals may become carriers and may infect other horses or species at any time during acute or remission periods and may remain infected for long periods.

310 (a) The history of chronic coughing during periods when the horse is stabled suggests that she is affected by COPD (chronic obstructive pulmonary disease). The acute respiratory distress demonstrated by the mare is probably due to acute small airway obstruction; this can occur in susceptible horses when they are suddenly exposed to an antigenic challenge (for example, when brought into a dusty box after a period at grass).
(b) The most important factor in the development of airway obstruction in most cases of COPD is exposure to organic dusts (especially mould spores) associated with hay, straw and stable dust. The first priority of treatment, therefore, is to remove the affected horse from its present environment into a 'clean' environment. Bronchodilator drugs should be used to relieve the bronchospasm; clenbuterol is probably the most widely used agent for this purpose. Other bronchodilators that can be used include theophylline and atropine. Corticosteroids are also useful for the treatment of acute airway obstruction; they act to stabilise lysosomal membranes, inhibit cellular migration, potentiate the actions of beta-2 receptor stimulants (such as clenbuterol) and increase the availability of cyclic AMP. Antibiotics may also be beneficial, since the clearance of bacteria from the lungs can be impeded in these cases.

311 (a) Solar margin fractures of the distal phalanx.

(b) These fractures may be incidental radiographic abnormalities, result from trauma, or occur in association with laminitis and rotation of the distal phalanx. It is possible that this animal has had a period of poor feeding followed by a period when it has been fed large amounts of concentrates to correct the problem of weight loss. This may have precipitated laminitis.

(c) Lateromedial projections of this animal's feet to establish whether there has been rotation of the distal phalanges.

312 (a) Abdominal radiography and abdominal ultrasound (to look for free peritoneal fluid and intestinal lesions such as intussusceptions), to determine the cause of the abdominal distention. If peritoneal fluid is present, abdominoparacentesis may be performed and the peritoneal fluid analysed. Blood cultures, serum IgG concentration, serum electrolytes, blood glucose, and thoracic radiographs are also indicated to determine the extent of disease in the foal.

(b) Enteritis/colitis, with or without a surgical lesion, such as torsion, displaced large bowel, intussusception; a surgical lesion alone; peritonitis. Uroperitoneum (with or without infection) is a less likely diagnosis (because of the increasing pain), but may accompany other conditions.

(c) Broad-spectrum antibiotics, and possibly plasma, depending on IgG levels. If the signs of pain worsen, or findings are suggestive of a surgical lesion, an exploratory laparotomy is indicated.

313 The complications of equine dental extraction can be summarised as failure to remove the correct tooth, the whole tooth and nothing but the tooth! Accurate diagnosis to identify which tooth, if any, is responsible for the clinical signs is essential before embarking on an extraction procedure. This requires a careful external examination of the head, a detailed oral inspection and radiographs using a suitable range of projections. Precise location of the trephine site over the root of the correct tooth is essential and can be aided by further radiographs using markers. Intraoperative catastrophes include:
- Fracture of the mandibular ramus.
- Damage to an adjacent root during repulsion.
- Rupture of parotid duct.
- Haemorrhage from palatine artery, linguofacial artery and vein.
- Damage to facial or infraorbital nerves.
- Trauma to nasolacrimal duct.
- Incomplete removal of tooth (*Figure 308*).
- Anaesthetic death.
  Postoperative complications:
- Dental sequestra.
- Sequestration of alveolar supporting bone.
- Oroantral fistula formation – failure of the oral defect to heal and repeated contamination of the maxillary sinus.
- Alveolar cementosis/osteitis.

314 (a) Aortic insufficiency. The character of the murmur is typical of aortic insufficiency. The murmur could be localised to the aortic/pulmonary area. The aorta is a midline structure and therefore murmurs of aortic insufficiency are often heard on both sides of the thorax. It is a common finding in the older horse.

(b) The M-Mode study shows vibration of the anterior mitral valve leaflet. This is caused by the regurgitant jet of blood striking the anterior mitral valve leaflet as the blood flows from the aorta back into the ventricle during diastole. This vibration is thought to be responsible for the buzzing quality of the murmur. The Doppler study shows the normal laminar flow of blood into the aorta during systole. This signal is displayed below the baseline. Disturbed flow is shown to be moving in the opposite direction during diastole. This disturbed flow represents the jet of aortic insufficiency. It is displayed above the baseline, but as the blood is moving at a higher velocity than can be displayed on the vertical axis, the signal has been wrapped around and is also visible below the baseline (signal aliasing).

(c) The pulse would be bounding in quality (hyperkinetic). The stroke volume of the ventricle increases due to an increase in preload caused by the aortic insufficiency. The diastolic pressure would decrease due to run-off of blood from the aorta into the ventricle. This would lead to a large systolic–diastolic pressure difference which would be palpable as an increase in amplitude of the pulse.

(d) Many horses with aortic insufficiency continue to perform well. If the work history of the horse is good it is obviously still able to maintain its cardiac output during exercise, and must be compensating adequately for the abnormal flow. If the condition progresses the horse may become unable to maintain its cardiac output during exercise and tiring and evidence of reduced performance would become apparent. If this occurs, the workload of the horse must be reduced or the animal retired from work.

Ultrasonography can be used to measure the left ventricular internal diameter. This gives an indication of the degree of volume overload. Periodic examination is advisable to monitor the progression of the condition. Aortic insufficiency is a common condition in the older horse and is due to degenerative changes in the aortic valve.

Ultrasonography will help to rule out other causes of aortic insufficiency, for example endocarditis and aortic valve prolapse. Changes in the work performance, changes in the quality of the murmur, an increase in the area of auscultation and the presence of a palpable thrill all indicate progression of the condition and a thorough investigation and reassessment must be made. Congestive cardiac failure secondary to aortic insufficiency is uncommon.

315 (a) An involucrum is present on the dorsal aspect of the third metatarsal bone just above the fetlock joint.
(b) Surgery to remove the sequestrum which is likely to be present (and was present) in this involucrum.

316 (a) Autoimmune.
(b) Skin biopsy is of value if intact vesicles or pustules can be sampled.
(c) Acanthocytes, neutrophils, eosinophils, and no intracellular bacteria.

317 Equine chorionic gonadotrophin (eCG – formerly known as pregnant mare serum gonadotrophin, PMSG) is produced by the endometrial cups which begin to develop at about 36 days after conception. By 40 days they are usually producing sufficient hormone for it to be detected by sensitive assays (e.g. radioimmunoassay). However, since mares which have not been tested for pregnancy before 40 days are unlikely to have been examined systematically during oestrus, the day of ovulation is usually usually unknown. Dating pregnancy from the last covering day can be erroneous so that blood sampling for eCG is best carried out after the 45th day in order to avoid inappropriate early testing. Between 45 and 60 days the vast majority of mares will

prove positive to any test used to detect eCG. After 60 days a small percentage of mares will become negative because some mares produce very little eCG but still remain pregnant. On average, eCG remains detectable until 120 days. However, earlier testing is more accurate, and more useful if a non-pregnant mare is detected and it is decided to cover her again during the same breeding season.

318 (a) *Parascaris equorum* – the eggs typically have a thick, brown roughened outer shell.

Strongyles – these cannot readily be differentiated to subfamily or species by morphological features. In these animals they are most likely to be cyathostome (small strongyle) eggs because the prepatent period of the large strongyles is longer than the approximate age of the foals.

(b) Both ascarids and strongyles are of clinical significance in these foals: infections may result in general illthrift/poor body condition or they may cause more specific signs.

P. equorum worms have an hepatic–pulmonary–intestinal migratory life-cycle. Signs of coughing and nasal discharge may occur during the pulmonary phase if large numbers of eggs are ingested, but the intestinal phase is the most pathogenic. Heavy infections commonly result in poorly grown or emaciated foals and occasionally small intestinal impaction or rupture may result from a balling-up of a mass of ascarid worms.

Strongyle infections may give rise to colic and/or diarrhoea. The colic is most probably associated with alterations in intestinal blood supply and, although classically associated with *Strongylus vulgaris*, it is possible that other strongyle species play a role in the pathogenesis of verminous colic. Strongyle infections may cause changes in faecal consistency but the specific entity of larval cyathostomiasis associated with small strongyle infections is not usually seen in foals.

319 (a) Phthisis bulbi (shrunken globe).
(b) Severe intraocular infection or inflammation, e.g. equine periodic ophthalmia.
(c) Enucleation.

320 (a) There is flattening of the caudal aspect of the humeral head and loss of congruity between the glenoid cavity of the scapula and the humeral head. The ventral angle of the scapula is modelled and has a rather irregular, fuzzy outline. There are poorly defined lucent areas in the subchondral bone of the caudal aspect of the distal scapula, surrounded by some sclerosis proximally.

(b) Osteochondrosis, infection. Given the history and clinical signs osteochondrosis is the most likely diagnosis. A greater degree of lameness would be expected in association with infection. The gross and cytological appearance of the synovial fluid, obtained when arthrocentesis was performed, should confirm that infection is not present. In association with osteochondrosis, total protein and white blood cell concentrations may be elevated but less than with infection.

(c) Carefully check other joints for evidence of synovial effusion. Osteochondrosis often affects more than one joint and in many joints will result in joint capsule distension, although this is rarely appreciated in the shoulder.

Radiograph the contralateral shoulder since the condition may be bilateral.

Lameness associated with osteochondrosis of the shoulder is usually improved by intra-articular analgesia but is rarely alleviated fully, therefore it is not necessary in most cases to look for an additional source of pain. The variable degree of lameness described in the history is typical.

(d) Surgical treatment by arthroscopic debridement of the lesions is likely to result in clinical improvement, although total resolution of lameness cannot be guaranteed. Prognosis is usually best in horses less than 18 months of age.

321 (a) The presence of a slight serous or catarrhal nasal discharge with some evidence of purulence might be indicative of a bacterial secondary infection condition subsequent to an upper respiratory tract virus infection. However, the inhalation of irritants such as smoke, chemicals or dust may be responsible.
(b) A full clinical examination is important to establish the existence or otherwise of pyrexia and other signs of respiratory tract infections. The temperature should be monitored several times daily. Tracheal sensitivity and local lymphadenopathy may be identified. The thorax should be auscultated carefully to determine the presence of adventitious lung sounds. Paired sera may be used to detect rising antibody titres to known viruses and pharyngeal swabs for virus isolation may be helpful. Haematology may help to confirm the presence of infection.
(c) In this case no fever was identified and the cause was found to be inhalation of smoke. Antibiotics may be useful if secondary bacterial infections are likely or are present. Most such secondary infections involve penicillin-sensitive streptococci. In this case the signs resolved spontaneously without recourse to therapeutic measures once the smoke source had been removed!

322 (a)
- Surgically remove all fibrous tissue without removing any tendons.
- Allow wound to granulate under the bandage.
- Apply a skin graft.
(b)
- Use a cradle.
- Apply repellant such as Cribox to the bandages.

323 (a) Lateral luxation of the patella.
(b) This can be a congenital or an acquired problem. In this case, it is likely to have been present since birth, since it is a small pony.
(c) The animal is likely to be a Shetland pony, or another miniature breed, in which the condition is congenital.

324 (a) Radiographic examination of the proximal metacarpal region and the carpus (remember the relationship between the middle carpal joint capsule and the palmar metacarpal nerves; subcarpal analgesia may alleviate pain associated with the middle carpal joint unless analgesia is effected by perineural analgesia of the lateral palmar nerve at the level of the distal row of carpal bones, prior to dividing into the palmar metacarpal nerves).

Ultrasonographic examination of the palmar metacarpal soft tissues, using a 7.5-MHz transducer, both with and without a stand-off.

Intra-articular of the middle carpal joint capsule (see above).
(b) This is a transverse ultrasonogram of the palmar metacarpal soft tissues obtained without a stand-off, approximately 4 cm distal to the distal aspect of the accessory carpal bone. There is a central large ill-defined hypoechoic area in the suspensory ligament.
(c) Proximal suspensory desmitis. Examine the contralateral limb ultrasonographically. Ill- or well-defined central hypoechoic areas, extending up to 1 cm longitudinally, may

be seen in the proximal part of the suspensory ligament of some clinically normal horses: these are usually fairly symmetrical bilaterally and are rarely as large as the lesion identified in this horse.
(d) Box rest and controlled walking exercise. Re-examine in 4–6 weeks. The prognosis is usually good in the absence of any associated radiographic abnormalities, provided that the horse is given adequate rest in the acute phase and there is improvement in the lesion identified ultrasonographically. *Figure 309* is the same horse 5 weeks later; the lesion is no longer detectable.

325 Preganglionic cervical sympathetic lesion, neck abscess.
This foal in *Figure 250* demonstrates Horner's syndrome and it can be reasonably assumed to be a preganglionic (i.e. brainstem, spinal cord or cervical sympathetic nerve) involvement because the sweating extends a considerable way down the neck, i.e. to the level of caudal aspect of C2. *Postganglionic* lesions result in sweating on the side of the face, but less sweating on the neck and only on the most cranial areas. With brainstem or spinal cord involvement other signs most often would be present.

326 (a) Although the navicular bone appears to be fractured, the apparent fracture line seems to extend beyond the distal horizontal border of the navicular bone and the foot is obviously unpacked.
(b) A better dorsal 60° proximal–palmarodistal oblique projection of the navicular bone is required, or, better still, a palmaroproximal–palmarodistal oblique view of the navicular bone. The latter confirmed the presence of a navicular fracture.
(c) The horse is always likely to go lame when it is worked. The owner should consider lag screw fixation of the navicular fracture.

327 (a)
● Intra-articular analgesia of the metatarsophalangeal joint – negative.
● Analgesia of the flexor tendon sheath – positive.
● Ultrasonographic examination of the plantar metatarsal soft tissues.
(b) The ultrasonogram is obtained using a stand off, either medial or lateral to the plantar midline. It is therefore not possible to assess properly the superficial and deep digital flexor tendons *per se* (these were normal). There is some echodense material subcutaneously; the sheath wall is thickened; there is some echodense material within the sheath suggestive of adhesion formation.
(c) Diagnosis: tenosynovitis.
Treatment: transection of the plantar annular ligament; exploration of the flexor tendon sheath and breakdown of adhesions. (The subcutaneous fascia was partially adhered to the skin; there was a considerable amount of vascular fibrous tissue subcutaneously incorporating the vascular bundle, which was displaced plantad. The tendon sheath wall proximal to the plantar annular ligament was very thickened. There were several large adhesions within the sheath which were transected.)
Postoperative care: controlled exercise and non-steroidal anti-inflammatory drugs as required.
Prognosis: guarded because of the degree of adhesion formation. The mare made a complete recovery.

328 A blood (serum) sample and a peritoneal fluid sample would be helpful in attempting to confirm a provisional diagnosis of uroperitoneum. The peritoneal fluid sample should be obtained by paracentesis abdominis. This procedure requires surgical preparation of a small area (perhaps 5 cm × 5 cm) at the most dependent point of the abdomen of the foal. The foal should then be restrained in the standing position, and a 1.5 in, 18 or 20 gauge needle should then be slowly advanced into the peritoneal cavity until peritoneal fluid is obtained.

The creatinine concentration in both the serum and the peritoneal fluid should be determined. If the peritoneal creatinine : serum creatinine ratio is greater than 2:1, it would support a diagnosis of uroperitoneum.

Measurement of serum K^+ values and determination of the K^+ creatinine clearance ratio are also indicated. Hyponatraemia, hypochloraemia and hyperkalaemia often occur in cases of uroperitoneum, and hyperkalaemia may be the most difficult of these entities to correct. Fluids with no K^+ (e.g. 5% or 10% glucose saline) should be used to restore electrolyte imbalance. Care should also be taken in the administration of mares' milk, which is high in K^+ (12 mEq/l) as foals have an inability to excrete excess K^+ when suckling, or being given, mares' milk.

329
- Dysphagia with abdominal pain.
- Pulse inappropriately high for the degree of pain.
- Gastric reflux which is very liquid, brownish green and has a specific smell.
- Snuffling respiratory noise from rhinitis and purulent material in nose.
- Behavioural changes, e.g. elephant tub stance (see *Figure 253*), backing into wall, slow mastication.
- Scanty, mucous-coated faeces.

330 (a) Septicaemia (most common organisms include *E. coli* and *Actinobacillus*).
(b) Complete blood count (CBC), fibrinogen and blood glucose determination could all provide supportive evidence. Positive blood cultures would be the only definitive ante-mortem diagnostic procedure.
(c) Broad-spectrum antibiotic therapy (for both Gram-positive and Gram-negative bacteria), fluid therapy to prevent circulatory collapse, intravenous plasma therapy (20–40 ml/kg) to boost serum IgG levels, and possibly, non-steroidal anti-inflammatory drugs, such as flunixin meglumine for its anti-endotoxic properties.

331
- Distension colic, i.e. a medical colic whose cause is undiagnosed and which recovers with conservative management. The presence of a large fetus makes rectal examination of the bowel difficult. Broodmares seem prone to large bowel displacements. Elimination of other possibilities and careful observation with time gives your diagnosis. Treat as for spasmodic colic.
- Colonic volvulus. Pregnant mares have a predisposition to colonic volvulus. Colic signs would be much more severe and per rectum horizontal distended large colon fills the caudal abdomen. Surgical intervention should be performed as quickly as possible.
- Premature foal. Vaginal and rectal examination will determine this. Deliver the foal as atraumatically as possible.
- Uterine torsion is a possibility with these signs. Palpate the broad ligaments of the uterus carefully. One broad ligament will be taut across the abdomen and the ovary

pulled away from the abdominal wall. The other will be pulled down its side of the abdomen. Per vaginam nothing abnormal may be seen unless the torsion is 180° or more. Treatment is by surgical correction.

- Uterine dorsoretroflexion is a rare complication characterised by acute colic and abdominal straining. The fetus is palpated inside the pelvic canal and dorsal to the vagina. Smooth muscle relaxants are given until it is possible to reposition the fetus per rectum.

332 (a) Maintain a sternal position, and provide supplementary oxygen nasal insufflation initially at 4–5 l/min. Further adjustments in flow rate are based on repeat arterial blood gas analysis; maintain Po_2 between 70 and 90 mmHg, if possible. Mechanical ventilation is not necessary at this time, but may be indicated if the condition worsens (increased effort of breathing, increased Pco_2).

(b) *In utero* acquired pneumonia; incomplete skeletal ossification.

(c) Broad-spectrum antibiotic therapy; provide colostrum by bottle or tube; intensive nursing care, including close monitoring of blood glucose and body temperature. Intravenous fluid therapy may be necessary.

(d) Short term, quite good, providing high-quality intensive respiratory and supportive care can be provided by a knowledgeable staff. Long-term prognosis is dependent on proper management of an immature musculoskeletal system, and on the prevention of secondary infections or complications. Adult body size may be slightly smaller than if the foal were born at term, but a late growth spurt may result in a normal-sized individual.

333 (a) Vaginal tunic and cremaster muscle.

(b) The vaginal tunic is related to the testis and once it and its contents have been identified, the surgeon knows where the testis is or whether it has been previously removed.

(c)

- An inguinally retained testis and its associated epididymis, vas deferens and blood vessels.
- A vas deferens and remains of blood vessels, usually terminating in a distal nub of fibrous tissue – this finding indicates that the horse has been castrated.
- A tail of epididymis attached to vas deferens and body of epididymis – the testis is within the abdomen as this is a case of incomplete abdominal retention.
- A vas deferens and a body of epididymis terminating in a distal nub of fibrous tissue – the testis is within the abdomen as this is a case of incomplete abdominal retention from which the epididymal tail has been removed, probably in the mistaken belief that it was a small or mis-shaped testis;
- The ligament of the tail of the epididymis which is derived from part of the fetal gubernaculum testis – the testis and the epididymis are both within the abdomen as this is a case of complete abdominal retention.

(d) The picture illustrates a large ligament of the tail of the epididymis within a vaginal tunic; the testis (which weighed 365g) and the epididymis were both removed at paramedian laparotomy.

334 (a) Rabies. Any progressive neurological condition which cannot be fully explained by another condition should arouse suspicion of rabies. Salivation, pharyngeal paralysis and progressive ascending hindlimb neurological deficits are the most consistent findings, and, generally, self-inflicted wounds occur at or near the site of the original injection of virus.

(b) Diagnosis may be confirmed by the finding at postmortem of characteristic Negri bodies in the hippocampus. Fluorescent antibody techniques may be used on smears made from conjunctival cells.

(c) Transmission from horses to man is uncommon but all in-contact persons should seek appropriate medical advice as soon as possible. Vaccination of other horses is effective and control of contact between the horses and possibly infected carnivores in particular may be practical.

335 (a) Uroperitoneum, most commonly a result of a ruptured urachus or urinary bladder.

(b) Peritoneal fluid analysis; measure creatinine in the sample and compare to serum levels. Also perform WBC count and cytology on the fluid, as infection of the umbilical remnants may be a complicating factor. If a laboratory is not available, new methylene blue injected into the urinary bladder, and retrieved from the peritoneal fluid, can also provide presumptive evidence of a disrupted urinary tract.

(c) 0.9% saline, with dextrose. If total CO_2 is low, sodium bicarbonate therapy may also be indicated.

336 (a) Nasogastric intubation.

(b) Such cases often have gastric distension due to the high obstruction. If this distension is not relieved prior to induction of anaesthesia, rupture of the stomach is likely. During anaesthesia such distension would severely compromise cardiovascular respiratory function by causing diaphragmatic splinting and pressure on the caudal vena cava, reducing venous return.

References

Cunha, T.J. (1991), *Horse Feeding and Nutrition*, 2nd edn, Academic Press, London.
Frape, D. (1986), *Equine Nutrition and Feeding*, Longman, Harlow.
McCarthy, G. (1987), *Pasture Management for Horses and Ponies*, Sheridan.
National Research Council (1989), *Nutrient Requirements of Horses*, 5th edn, Wiley and Washington National Academy Press.

INDEX

Numbers refer to question and answer numbers.